W9-CED-561

Important Telephone Numbers

Emergency Room _____

_____

Poison Control Center _____

_____

Ambulance _____

_____

Family Doctor _____

_____

Specialist _____

_____

Specialist _____

_____

Dentist _____

_____

Dentist's Emergency No. _____

_____

Hospital No. _____

_____

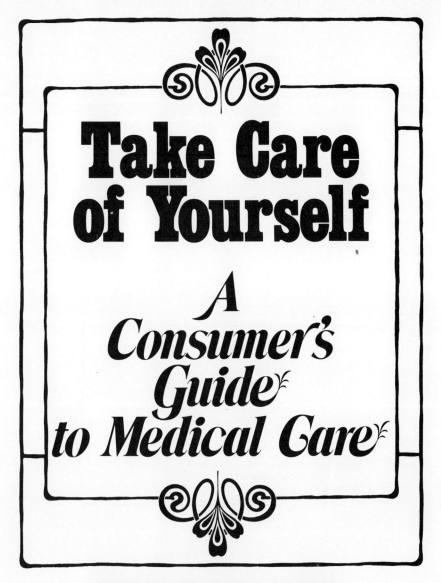

Take Care of Yourself

A Consumer's Guide to Medical Care

Donald M. Vickery, M.D.

James F. Fries, M.D.

ADDISON-WESLEY PUBLISHING COMPANY

READING, MASSACHUSETTS • MENLO PARK, CALIFORNIA
LONDON • AMSTERDAM • DON MILLS, ONTARIO • SYDNEY

Library of Congress Cataloging in Publication Data

Vickery, Donald M.
  Take care of yourself.

  Includes index.
  1. Medicine, Popular.   2. Medical care.
I. Fries, James F., joint author.   II. Title.
RC81.V5   616'.024   76–1378

ISBN 0-201-02401-2 H
ISBN 0-201-02402-0 P
ISBN 0-201-02403-9 S

Fifth printing, July 1978

Copyright © 1976 by Addison-Wesley Publishing Company, Inc. Philippines copyright 1976 by Addison-Wesley Publishing Company, Inc.
All rights reserved. No part of this publication may be reproduced, stored in a retrieval system, or transmitted, in any form or by any means, electronic, mechanical, photocopying, recording, or otherwise, without the prior written permission of the publisher. Printed in the United States of America. Published simultaneously in Canada. Library of Congress Catalog Card No. 76–1378

0-201-02403-9
FGHIJK-HA-798

Preface

Two new developments in medical care now make it possible for consumers to play more active roles in taking care of themselves. Without these new developments—the training of physician-assistants and the growing use of the computer in medicine—this book could not have been written.

First, the need for more medical personnel has resulted in training programs for para-medical professionals. These physician-assistants can effectively handle many common health problems so that doctors can concentrate on more complicated medical conditions. The training programs for physician-assistants have provided the first logical rules for deciding when a patient should see a doctor.

Second, the computer is being used more widely in medicine. After analyzing the problems of diagnosis, treatment, and referral, computer programmers have developed a way to describe the medical thinking process. What they have devised are the "flow-charts" or "instruction charts" similar to the ones in Section II of this book.

Both authors are involved in these developments. At Johns Hopkins, Dr. Fries produced the first instruction chart for medical diagnosis in 1970. Later, he worked with the Robert Wood Johnson Clinical Scholar Program at Stanford to examine consumer education and cost effectiveness in medicine and to use computer analysis to dissect some of the essential ingredients of medical decisions.

In the meantime, at Ft. Belvoir, Virginia, Dr. Vickery was developing flow charts and manuals for an Army training program of physician-assistants called Project AMOS. Later, as Director of the Reston, Virginia, Medical Center, he established "patient education" as a formal course to help the local citizens to become informed medical consumers. He also developed a "triage manual" which used the flow-chart method to help nurses and receptionists refer and schedule patients.

Thanks to these two new developments—physician-assistants and the computer—consumers can have the information they need to make sound medical decisions for themselves and their families. That is what this book is all about.

Reston, Va.   D.M.V.
Stanford, Calif.   J.F.F.
February, 1976

Acknowledgments

Many individuals have contributed concepts, insights, review or criticism to this book. We are grateful for the observation that when a typical patient encounters a typical doctor, there is only fifty-fifty chance of benefit to the patient, for the gentle admonition that the good physician is like a wise grandmother who knows little of medical science but can tell who is sick and who is not, for a fictional clinic with treatment based solely upon the height of the fever, and to the social critic who noted that healing commonly occurs in spite of physician efforts. The synthesis of these themes is our responsibility.

We gratefully acknowledge the help of: Dr. John Beck, Lewis Carroll, Dr. Theresa Del Presto, Dr. Anthony De Paola, Dr. Leonard Eppard, Joseph Heller, Dr. Halsted Holman, Dr. Oliver Wendell Holmes, Dr. Robert Huntley, Dr. Julius Krevans, Dr. Kurt Lederer, Dr. Paul Lairson, Dr. John Lyles, Dr. Dennis McShane, Dr. Donald Mitchell, Dr. William Osler, Dr. Louis Rittlemeyer, Dr. David Rogers, Dr. Ralph Rosenthal, George Bernard Shaw, John Slane, Dr. Michael Soper, Kurt Vonnegut, Jr., Dr. John Wasson, and Dr. William Watson.

Sarah and Shelley helped too—a lot.

Manuscript preparation would not have been possible without the yeoman efforts of Carolyn Hinkle, Bonnie Obrig, and Colette Marshall.

Our thanks also go to our editors who encouraged us to tell seldom-told-tales, and who refrained, sometimes with difficulty, from saying: "you can't say that."

To Our Readers

This book is powerful medicine. It can be of great help to you. The medical advice is as sound as we can make it. But it will not always work. Like advice from your doctor or nurse, it will not always prove successful. This is our problem: if we don't give you direct advice we can't help you. If we do, we will sometimes be wrong. So here are some qualifications: If you are under the care of a physician and receive advice contrary to this book, follow the physician's advice; the individual characteristics of your problem can then be taken into account. If you have an allergy or a suspected allergy to a recommended medicine, check with your doctor, at least by phone. With any medicine, read the label directions carefully; instructions vary from year to year and you should follow the latest. And if your problem persists, beyond a reasonable period, you should usually see a doctor.

Contents

7

The Home Pharmacy
43

8

Avoiding Medical Fraud
67

Section II

The Patient and the Common Complaint

73

A

How to Use This Section
75

B

Emergencies
77

C

Common Injuries
81

D

Poisons
105

E

Ears, Nose, and Throat
109

F

Common Skin Problems
129

G

Childhood Rashes With Fever
159

The Digestive Tract
217

The Urinary Tract
229

N

For Women Only
237

O

Sexual Problems
251

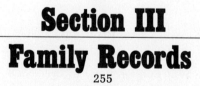

Section III

Family Records
255

Index
263

Introduction

You can do more for your health than your doctor can. As an enlightened medical consumer, you can save money and time, and provide for the best possible medical care for yourself and your family. You can learn to treat many medical problems at home. And you can learn to recognize when it's important to get to a doctor or hospital. You can learn how to cut the high costs of medicine. And you can learn to choose the right physician and medical facility for your family. This book will show you how.

Many people think that all illness must be treated at a physician's office or at a hospital. They go to doctors rather than relying on remedies which worked perfectly well in less complex times. The average family of four now sees the doctor more than 12 times each year at an average cost of over $35 per visit for services, tests, and drugs—that's over $400 a year!

Demand for physicians' services has steadily grown. In 1973, there were 325 *million* more doctor visits than in 1964. This greater demand contributes to longer waiting lines, less time with the doctor, increased physician charges, and higher medical-insurance premiums. Most of these visits are made for relatively minor medical problems. In our national quest for a symptom-free existence, as many as 70 percent of visits to the doctor have been termed "unnecessary." The competent physician's response to these visits is either to reassure the patient or to advise measures which are available without prescription.

Clearly, if appropriate information is available, much of this medical care can be handled at home. To accomplish this, you need to be able to distinguish minor problems from those which require a visit to the doctor. It is our purpose, here, to provide you with that information.

This book outlines a method for you to make sound judgments about most of the medical problems which you will encounter. It is based on a system of rules, which provide step-by-step approaches to the most common health problems. These guidelines either indicate a program of self-treatment or suggest a visit or telephone call to the doctor.

1

We have designed this book as a practical resource—a do-it-yourself guide to medical care. We hope you will keep it handy for ready reference. You can use the page at the beginning of the book to keep emergency telephone numbers and the Family Record section (Section III) to record immunizations and medical histories for your family.

As a patient, you are also a client, a customer, a consumer, and a critic. Section I of this book provides practical information for these roles. Read these chapters first; they provide a solid health-information background to help you make the right medical decisions for yourself and your family. You'll learn about:

Your habits: how they directly affect your health.

Preventive medicine: the myth of the annual check-up, the limitations of multiphasic screening, the importance of early treatment, and new information on some immunizations—How often do we need them?

How to choose the right doctor: understanding the different types of doctors, medical practices, and payment systems; tip-offs to poor medical service, and guidelines for selecting the right doctor for you and your family.

The office visit: what medical procedures to expect and how you can actively participate in your own diagnosis and treatment.

How to find the right medical facility: hospitals and when to use them, emergency rooms, convalescent homes, and free clinics.

Hints on reducing the high cost of drugs: how your physician and pharmacist can help you save money.

Your home pharmacy: how to stock it with the most effective medicines for minor medical problems; hints on reading labels, dosage, and possible side effects for a variety of over-the-counter medicines.

Medical fraud: how some common sense can save you money and help you avoid medical hustles.

Section II of this book provides specific guidance for 68 of the most common medical problems. We have designed this section so that it is easy to use. First, you identify your primary symptom, for instance: a cough, a stomachache, a cut finger, chest pain, poison ivy, etc. Then, to find discussion of your problem, look it up in the Table of Contents or the Index.

Each of the medical problems in Section II includes a general discussion of the complaint, suggestions on how to treat it at home, and information on what to expect at the doctor's office—if you go. The charts which accompany each problem provide step-by-step instructions to help you decide if you should use home treatment or if you should seek medical advice. No medicine suggested in Section II should be used without knowledge of its dosage and its side effects. Most medicines are discussed in Chapter 7.

Using the guidelines in this book, you can save time and money and ease our overloaded health-care system. More important, by learning to identify the significance of medical problems, you can ensure that professional medical care is obtained when it is needed. With this information, you can take good care of yourself and your family.

Section

I

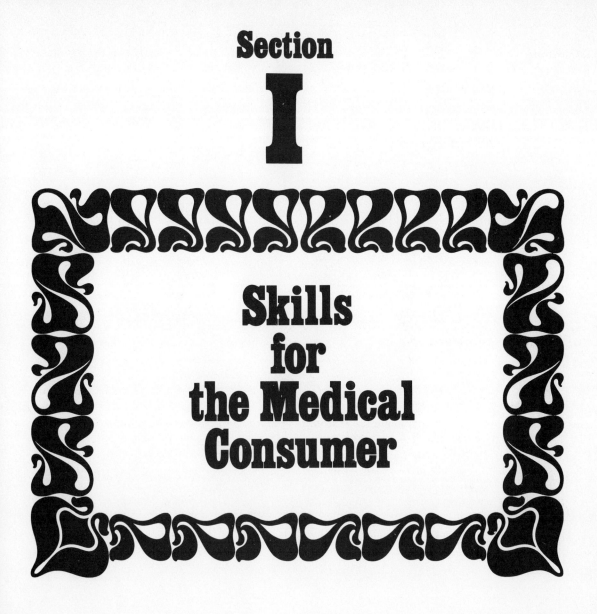

Skills
for
the Medical
Consumer

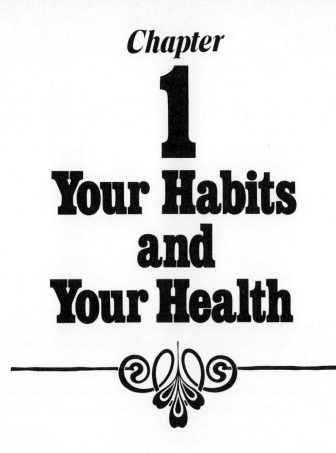

Chapter
1
Your Habits and Your Health

For the most part, your health is up to you. You can do much more than any physician to maintain your own good health and wellbeing.

With the exception of those diseases which are prevented by immunizations, surprisingly few diseases can be *prevented* by the physician. On occasion, the physician may detect that you have tuberculosis, high blood pressure, or an early and treatable cancer. Diagnostic tools as the chest x-ray, the blood pressure cuff, and the Pap smear may be used to make such a diagnosis. In these instances, medical treatment is able to significantly contribute to your long-term health. Unfortunately, such instances are rare. For the majority of diseases, it makes little difference when they are recognized because there is no effective way to prevent their progression.

On the other hand, the elements of health controlled by the patient affect every individual's well-being. Your doctor's examination of your heart will not prevent a heart attack, but you can decrease your chances of a heart attack by simple measures of diet and exercise. You don't really need a physician to remind you that alcohol acts to destroy the liver and stomach lining or that you can avoid lung diseases if you quit smoking tar-laden cigarettes, or that fat people have more health problems than do slim ones.

If we could eliminate all unhealthy habits, what would happen? Lung cancer and emphysema would almost completely disappear, death due to all cancers would decrease by 25 percent, cirrhosis of the liver would become a rare disease; peptic ulcers, gastritis, and esophagitis (inflammation of the stomach and esophagus) would decrease in frequency; massive upper G.I. hemorrhage (bleeding from the stomach) would be unusual; pancreatitis (inflammation of the pancreas) would be rare; elevated blood pressure would be less common; atherosclerosis (hardening of the arteries) would decrease in frequency; and accidental injuries would become less frequent. Without the help of the patient, medicine can make no such promises. Let's examine some habits that directly affect our health:

COFFIN NAILS

Cigarette smoking *is* hazardous to your health. Physicians define "pack years" as the number of packs smoked per day multiplied by the number of years you have smoked. For example, if you smoked two packs per day for five years, you are a ten pack-year smoker. For each pack-year which you smoke, your life expectancy is decreased by about one month. A heavy smoker, smoking two packs daily for 30 years, or 60 pack-years, has decreased life expectancy by 5 years.

Just as important, the last years of a cigarette smoker are not a thing of grace and beauty. Tortuous wheezing, swollen purple lips, and near-suffocation when you're resting mark this condition. In medical jargon, the late-stage cigarette smoker is called a "blue bloater." Fortunately, however, present evidence suggests that the ex-cigarette smoker can improve life expectancy, although not back to that of the nonsmoker. Pipes and cigars, *when not inhaled,* are less hazardous and account for only a fraction of the problems of inhaled cigarette smoking.

THE TWO-MARTINI LUNCH

Alcohol is enjoyed by the great majority of individuals in the United States. In moderation, it may improve circulation, reduce blood pressure, and act as a mild and safe sedative. However, some 10 percent of our population have serious drinking problems. These people make up 20 percent of our hospitalized patients. Typically, they are ill with a variety of serious problems. Liver disease, ulcer disease, bleeding from the bowel, and vitamin deficiencies are among the most frequent. Sometimes they show signs of mental derangement, or exhibit the spectacular "delirium tremens"—the "DT's" or "the shakes." Alcohol is high in calories. With heavy drinking, there is a tendency to eat less nutritional food. This can result in a variety of nutritional problems as well as cirrhosis of the liver.

Treatment of the alcoholic continues to be a frustrating, often unsuccessful venture. Within the medical community, enthusiasm waxes and wanes for a wide variety of treatment methods. Nonmedical organizations, especially Alcoholics Anonymous, enjoy a success rate which at least equals that of any "medical" method. Associated organizations, such as Al Anon, which work with the families of alcoholics, also show great promise.

DRUGS

The history of humankind has shown that all drugs can be used to excess, with harmful consequences. This is known to be true for the major drugs of our society: alcohol, nicotine, and caffeine. Evidence suggests strongly that this situation holds also for the drugs of the "youth culture" and for the medically prescribed "happiness pills" of their parents.

Marijuana is a rather mild drug with a soothing effect. However, experiments indicate that large amounts of marijuana used over a long period of time may cause genetic damage in animals. Its effects on humans are not fully known. Thus while marijuana may not prove to be as harmful as alcohol, it is impossible, at present, to say what its hazards may be. Amphetamines and "speed" stimulate the body, creating an illusion of extra energy, but they almost certainly increase some forms of heart disease by constricting the small blood vessels. The "hard" drugs and narcotics (such as heroin, cocaine, morphine, demerol, and methadone) have potential for fatal overdose, and addiction invariably leads to social degeneration of the user. A large fraction of crimes, both violent and nonviolent, are related to these drugs; not because the user is directly influenced by the drug, but because money must be obtained to buy more.

The indiscriminate introduction of tranquilizers and other mood-changing agents into general medicine has been viewed with dismay by many observers, including ourselves. Many of these drugs now top the list of prescription medications; they are prescribed more frequently than any other drugs. In the language of the street, they can be divided into "uppers" and "downers."

The "uppers" are the amphetamines. They are often prescribed in a misguided attempt to help the patient to lose weight. They do not assist in weight reduction, except temporarily, and studies attempting to demonstrate their effectiveness as weight aids have failed. They cause severe mood changes, tightening of the small arteries, and impose an extra strain on the heart. These drugs have been used in the athletic arena by trainers and players, because they create the illusion of physical prowess. Careful studies in track-and-field events, where direct measurement of performance is possible, show that they neither help nor hinder performance of events such as the hundred-yard dash or the mile, but have a tendency to impair performance in events requiring coordination, such as the hurdles and pole vault.

The "downers" are even more popular, and for even less understandable reasons. They are frequently prescribed when a patient reports "nervousness" or "anxiety." That is, they are given for symptoms reflecting difficulty in coping. But these drugs further impair the ability to cope with the immediate environment! One standard tablet of most of these medications (such as Librium, Valium) is roughly equivalent, as a sedative, to a one ounce alcoholic drink. Most would agree that taking one or two drinks four times a day is not a successful way to solve life's problems.

Sedatives are also given to "help" patients sleep. Insomnia is a troublesome complaint, but it is not a disease. The body's instinct for restorative sleep is extremely powerful; when sleep is truly needed, it is demanded by the body. In many adults, four to six hours of sleep may be perfectly ample. In some individuals, a feeling of poor sleep for one night is followed by an early bedtime the second night, with periods of wakefulness that night leading to an impression of poor sleep, which stimulates an even earlier bedtime the following night. True insomnia requiring medical treatment is very rare. Sedatives are seldom necessary.

If you do use sedatives, you or your child or your neighbor may die of an overdose of them. They affect enzymes in the liver, leading to complications when other drugs are used at the same time. They may carry over into a morning hangover, and they increase the chance that your children won't listen to you when you tell them about the evils of their drugs.

Drugs are chemicals. In the bloodstream, the drugs which you swallow react with other drugs or with various chemicals already made by your body. If several drugs are being taken at once, the complexity of these interactions is such that no physician understands them. Many symptoms and side-effects may come from a medication or a combination of medications taken. It is now estimated that between 10 and 20 percent of hospital admissions are the direct result of complications of prescription drugs. The majority of drugs which cause these reactions are medically *optional* and are *not* required to maintain the health of the patient. Even common laxatives have been associated with a number of medical complications. Medications do not make you healthy so don't look for health in a pill bottle.

THE FAT OF THE LAND

Overeating is the most frequent of the American vices, costing the average citizen a year of life. Insurance company figures indicate that once you are 10 pounds over your ideal weight, each additional pound costs you a month of your life.

It is less well known that the fat individual doesn't even get to eat significantly more than his thin counter-part. A day's food for an average individual represents about one pound of body weight. If you fast for a day, you lose a pound of flesh. If you eat double, you gain a pound. A fat person may gain weight at a rate of 10 pounds each year; in a few years this rate of accumulation will result in an extremely obese individual. The ten extra pounds represent the intake of only ten extra days worth of food during the course of the year. Thus, in 365 days, the fat individual has eaten enough food for 375 days. This represents less than 3 percent difference between an appropriate diet and a diet leading to extreme obesity; hardly enough to increase the pleasure of eating. Some people never have a weight problem; others are less fortunate and are constantly plagued. We respect the difficulty of this condition, but it has a personal and not a medical solution.

It is not clear why fat people die sooner. We do know that they have higher blood pressure and higher blood fats. They develop hardening of the arteries at earlier ages. They have more surgical complications, particularly with abdominal operations.

A very few people have glandular troubles which cause their weight problem, but, for most of us, there are no good reasons for being overweight. Excuses will not prevent the consequences. You must decide your own priorities. "Overworked and overweight" go together only if you let them. The vast majority of us must choose between calories and complications, between early diet and early demise.

FITNESS

Without exercise, the muscles get flabby. The bones become brittle. The heart muscle becomes soft; in medical terms, "cardiac reserve" is lost. The weakened heart muscle is less able to respond to the needs of stressful situations. Improved muscle tone and increased activity strengthens bones and ligaments as well as muscles.

No exact figures document the extent to which exercise is important for life-expectancy. However, most authorities believe that lack of physical activity in the United States accounts for much of our poor record in longevity. Nearly everyone newly involved in a regular exercise program feels more energetic. The ability to withstand stress such as surgery or heart attacks is directly related to the physical condition of the body. Walking, jogging, swimming, and bicycling are easy and pleasurable ways to put regular physical activity back into your life.

ACCIDENTS

The fastening of an automobile seatbelt is seldom considered as medical treatment. Seatbelts, interlock devices, speed limits, and stop signs are frequently considered bureaucratic nuisances which impede the freedom of the individual. However, preventive medicine includes eliminating the major causes of death and suffering. If you are between the ages of 15 and 35, the most likely cause of your death in the next year is an accident. The majority of these deaths occur on the highway. At this age, you can for the most part forget about cancer, strokes, heart attacks, and other major medical problems. Beware instead the show-off, the drunk, and the harming of your own passengers. Young Americans who die on the highway usually perish by the hand of another young American.

THE SELF-DESTRUCTION SYNDROMES

Cigarettes, alcohol, drugs, fat, inactivity, and accidents—each of these subjects represents a form of suicide. The combined effect of these factors can take two years or more off your life expectancy. You can live longer and feel better by employing certain restraints in your life style. Absolute prohibition of activities is not required, but application of some discipline is necessary. It is important to remember that each of these health factors accumulates its effects. Thus, the longer you smoke, the longer you permit obesity, the longer you lack exercise, and the percentage of time you ignore your seatbelts affects the probability of death or disability. Stopping at any time is beneficial. Moderation rather than elimination is the crucial concept.

Be honest with yourself. Avoid excuses. "I hardly eat a thing." "I don't smoke the cigarettes all the way." "I never drink before lunch time." "I can handle it." "The only exercise I want is bending my elbow." "I don't use the seat belt because I want to be able to get out of the car in case of an accident." Such statements are excruciatingly self-revealing. It is embarrassing to hear them stated by apparently intelligent people. They demonstrate a painful lack of insight and self-knowledge.

How can you specifically approach the task of conquering a habit? Unfortunately, only by hard work! Avoid self-deception. Write things down. Keep diaries. Make charts. Set goals. Weigh yourself frequently. (Do it at the same time of day and on the same scale.) After initially losing a desired amount of weight, set narrow limits and continue the discipline. Change eating habits, but don't torture yourself. When possible, decrease the number of eggs, fatty meats, butter, and ice cream. Stop buying cigarettes. (Consider a pipe or cigars.) Consider beer and wine instead of hard liquor. Find a pleasurable exercise, and practice it regularly.

Decide to make permanent changes in your life. Crash diets, going "on the wagon," and spurts of severe physical activity are all poor practice. When you exercise beyond your conditioning, you stress the heart. If your weight goes from high to low and back again like a yo-yo, it is probably more harmful to your heart and arteries than if you maintained a stable (yet higher) weight. The spree drinker passes from unconsciousness to shaking and back again with regularity.

You are the patient. It is *your* life and *your* responsibility. Define for yourself those health goals which are important to you and to your family. Define a solid and workable program to approach these goals, and plan to maintain that program for the rest of your life. You will live longer, feel better, and have more energy for family and friends.

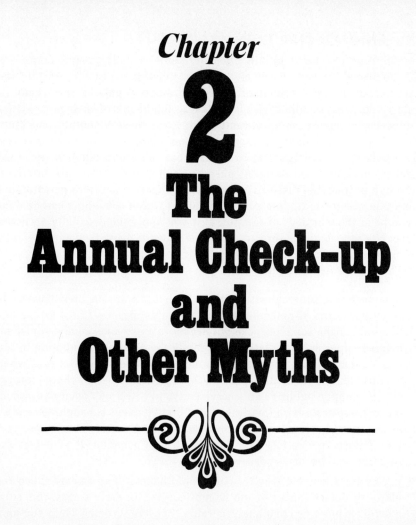

Chapter
2
The Annual Check-up and Other Myths

Medicine has been criticized for being "crisis-oriented." Often, the major emphasis of medical care has been on intensive treatment of the crisis rather than on measures for maintaining health and preventing the crisis. However, more and more interest is now focusing on preventive medicine and health maintenance. The idea of preventive medicine includes these four health care measures:

- The checkup or periodic health examination
- Multi-phasic screening
- Early treatment
- Immunizations and other public health measures

The following discussion will help you to distinguish those concepts which are important from those which you may more safely ignore.

THE ANNUAL CHECKUP

The "routine checkup" is still urged by some schools, camps, employers, and the armed services. Curiously, doctors never go to each other for "routine checkups." The "executive physical," made popular a few years ago by large corporations that wished to insure the health of their most critical employees, is slowly being discontinued. Even these elaborate check-ups, which take several days, do not detect early and treatable diseases with any regularity. It is important to realize that the organization requesting a medical checkup has a different purpose than you do. *They are interested in finding untreatable diseases which might affect your future performance; you are interested in finding conditions about which something can be done.* If you heed the warnings of Chapter 1, if you apply the discipline necessary to regulate your habits, there are very few advantages to be gained from the "routine checkup."

There are a few exceptions, and you should bear them in mind:

- Skin tests for tuberculosis (PPD or Tine Test) are an inexpensive and effective means of detecting exposure to this disease. Chest x-rays may be used for the same purpose but are more expensive, cumbersome, and involve exposure to radiation. (Although the amount of radiation in routine x-rays is small, your general policy should be to avoid x-rays whenever possible). Frequently, these tests are available free of charge through city or county public health services. While it is customary to recommend these tests on a yearly basis, a less frequent schedule (every 3–5 years) is probably adequate *unless* you have definitely been exposed to tuberculosis or live in an area in which it is common. If your test was negative, and becomes positive, check with your doctor.

- If you are a woman over 25, you should have a "Pap smear" taken regularly to detect cancer of the womb (cervix). In early stages, this slow-growing cancer is completely curable. See For Women Only for more information on Pap smears. If you are a woman over 25, you should also practice breast self-examination every month, and should check out any suspicious lumps with your physician. Mammography (a special breast x-ray) is not recommended as a screening procedure except for those who already have had a breast tumor or who have a family history of breast cancer. This procedure is expensive and not always reliable.

- A test for glaucoma (a treatable disease which can cause blindness) should be done after age forty if there is a family history of glaucoma.

- Urinalysis, urine cultures, tests for blood in the stool after age 30, sigmoidoscopy after age 50 are screening procedures which are ordered by many physicians. They have value in particular circumstances. Take your doctor's advice on these.

- During adult life, it is advisable to have a blood pressure check made at least every year or so. This measurement can easily be done by a nurse, physician's assistant, or nurse's aide. A full examination is not required.

Congratulations: You just saved an executive examination costing $300. The important elements of elaborate examinations are the blood pressure check, tuberculosis screening, breast examination and pap-smear tests for women, and glaucoma tests when a family history is present.

MULTIPHASIC SCREENING

Multiphasic screening simply means that many laboratory tests are performed in an attempt to find an abnormality which is not readily apparent. Some multiphasic screening programs will perform fifty or more different tests, including blood studies, urinalysis, x-rays, electrocardiograms, and other procedures. With automation, these many tests can be performed surprisingly quickly and economically. You can sometimes have nearly a hundred tests performed for less cost than that of a physical examination.

As a rule, however, we do not recommend multiphasic screening.

Experience with these screening systems over several years has shown that many laboratory abnormalities can be detected but that hardly any problems which need immediate treatment are found. Doctors have been required to follow up on the minor laboratory abnormalities, increasing cost and worry to the patient. Some medical administrators have remarked that the real purpose of multiphasic screening is to reassure the "worried well," at the lowest possible cost. In other words, it is less expensive to send a patient a letter stating that the tests are all negative and that health is perfect than it is for a physician to examine a patient and say the same thing. Thus, multiphasic screening procedures have become a means of mass reassurance.

It is now generally admitted that screening is justified only for those individual tests which potentially detect important and treatable illness. These are the same items mentioned earlier: Blood pressure evaluation, Pap smears, breast examination, and skin tests or x-rays for tuberculosis. Mammography of the breasts, eye testing for glaucoma, and testing the stool for blood are indicated for high-risk patients. In many settings, the blood pressure is the only truly important measurement.

EARLY TREATMENT

The best health maintenance strategy is to seek medical care promptly whenever a truly important complaint or finding occurs. If you find a lump in your breast, if you have unexplained weight loss, if you have begun to cough up blood, if you have been running fevers for more than a week; then you should seek medical attention without undue delay. These are not emergencies, but do indicate that attention should be sought within a very few days. Many times, nothing will be seriously wrong. On other occasions, however, an early cancer, tuberculosis, or other treatable disease may be located.

The guidelines of this book can help you select those instances in which you should seek medical care. In many cases, you can take care of yourself with home treatment. However, it is important to be ready when professional care is needed.

To insure timely treatment, think things through ahead of time. If you do need emergency care, where will you go? To an emergency hospital? To the emergency room of a general hospital? To the on-call physician of a local medical group? Rarely will you need emergency services. But the time that you do require them is not the time to begin wondering how to do it. If you have a routine problem which requires medical care, where are you going to go? Is there a near-by doctor who is available? Who has your necessary medical records on file? Define the methods you will use to obtain medical care before you need them.*

IMMUNIZATIONS

A final concept of preventive medicine concerns immunizations and other public health measures. These measures have far greater impact on health in developed nations than do the personal health services provided by physicians. Only a few years ago, smallpox, cholera, malaria, diphtheria, tetanus, and yellow fever killed entire populations. Now, these diseases are effectively controlled by immunization and other measures in this country.

There is a curious result of these health care measures: since no one in the country has smallpox, there is no one to catch it from, so smallpox vaccination is no longer routinely recommended. From the public health standpoint this is controversial; if the population does not remain vaccinated, a new epidemic could sweep the country. But in the absence of an epidemic there is little need to *repeat* immunization for this disease. Indeed, many immunizations do not need to be repeated nearly as frequently as was previously felt. Thus, for adults who have had their basic series of tetanus injections, tetanus boosters are not required more often than every 10 years. In many patients, smallpox and diphtheria immunizations last for life. With the increasing rarity of these diseases, the problems of side effects from the inoculations have become as great as the risk of illness in some instances.

Therefore, keep a careful record of your immunizations in the back of this book. Do not allow yourself to be re-inoculated just because you face a requirement for immunization and you have lost proof of previous immunization. If you haven't had a tetanus shot in the past 10 years ask your

---

* Chapter 3, "Finding The Right Physician," and Chapter 5, "Choosing the Right Medical Facility," will help you answer these questions.

physician for a routine shot when you are in the office for some other purpose. You can save a trip and be protected for another 10 years. In general, don't seek out the optional inoculations. Flu shots, for instance, are only partially effective and often cause a degree of illness themselves. They are recommended only for the elderly and for those with severe lung diseases.

Finally, here is a summary of what you need to remember about preventive medicine:

- You don't need "checkups" except for a very few specific tests. Blood pressure, Pap smears, periodic self-examination of the breasts, tuberculosis screening measures, and testing for glaucoma continue to make sense. Most of these procedures can be obtained through public health departments at city or county expense. Take your doctor's advice concerning the need for a urinalysis, urine culture, tests of the stool for blood, or sigmoidoscopy.

- Elaborate physical examinations and multi-phasic screening may worry you unnecessarily by discovery of trivial abnormalities.

- You should investigate methods of obtaining medical care *before* the need for care arises.

- You should be immunized according to recommended schedules, but you seldom need "boosters" in adult life.

If you follow these general procedures and if you control your living habits as discussed in the last chapter, then you are well on the way to taking care of yourself.

Chapter
3
Finding the Right Physician

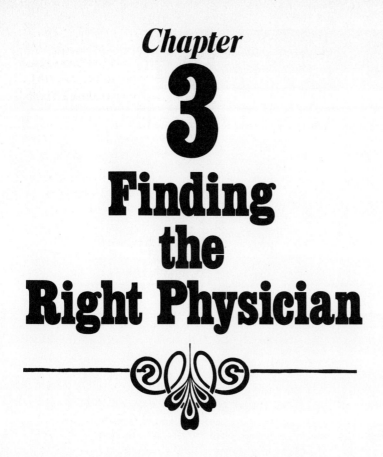

Who is the right doctor for you? There are all kinds of physicians, and the distinctions among them can be extremely confusing. This chapter is designed to help you understand the different types of doctors and how they run their medical practices. We provide you with some guidelines to help you choose the right doctor for you and your family.

To identify the different types of physicians, look at the three levels of specialization in Fig. 1. First, there are generalists or primary care physicians. Second, there are specialists in internal medicine, surgery, pediatrics, obstetrics and gynecology, or psychiatry. And finally, there are a large number of subspecialties which are directly related to one of the specialties.

THE FAMILY DOCTOR

The primary care physician, or generalist, is commonly called a general practitioner, GP, or family doctor. Often, a specialist in internal medicine or pediatrics will serve as a primary care physician. Family doctors may refer patients to other physicians but they seldom receive referrals.

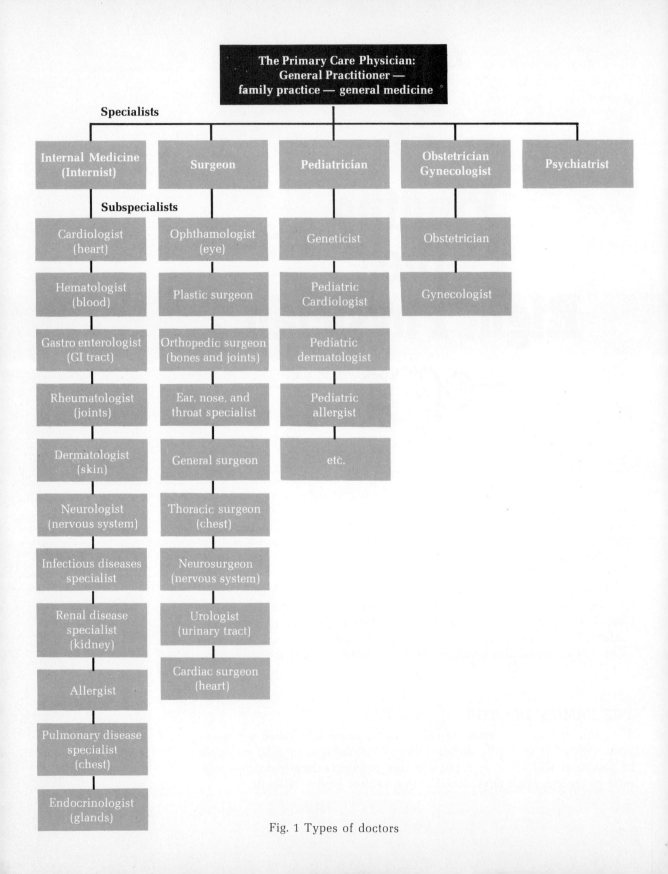

Fig. 1 Types of doctors

These physicians represent the initial contact between the patient and the medical establishment. They accept responsibility for the continued care of a patient or a family and perform a wide variety of services. Usually, they have had some training in internal medicine, pediatrics, and gynecology. In the past, they performed both major and minor surgery; but in recent years, this practice has become much less common, and the family doctor will usually refer major surgical problems to surgeons. Obstetrics and gynecology, the female specialties, are not always handled by general practitioners.

Family doctors serve as the quarterbacks of the medical system and may direct and coordinate a variety of activities they do not perform personally. Next to the patient, the generalist makes the most important decisions in medicine by determining the nature and severity of the problem and what approach to its solution should be used.

THE SPECIALISTS

The five major clinical specialties are internal medicine, surgery, pediatrics, obstetrics and gynecology, and psychiatry. There are other specialties such as radiology, clinical pathology, and anesthesiology; these are not included in our chart because the patient seldom goes directly to such physicians. The largest specialty is internal medicine. Physicians may refer to this specialty as "medicine," and to its practitioner as an "internist." The internist is sometimes confused with the "intern." An *intern* is a recent medical school graduate undergoing hospital apprenticeship in any area of medicine; an *internist* is a specialist in internal medicine usually having completed three or more years of training after graduation from medical school. Each of the other specialties has a similar length of training.

THE SUBSPECIALISTS

Subspecialties have developed within the major specialty areas; some are listed in Fig. 1. In internal medicine, there is a specialist for nearly every organ system. Thus, the heart has its cardiologists, the skin its dermatologists, the nervous system its neurologists, the kidney its renal disease specialists, and so forth. Within surgery, different types of operations have defined the specialties of particular surgeons. The ophthalmologist performs surgery on the eyes; the ear, nose, throat specialist (ENT) on those areas, the thoracic surgeon in the chest, and the cardiac surgeon on the heart. The general surgeon operates in the abdominal cavity as well as other areas.

Within pediatrics, specialties have developed similar to those within adult internal medicine. In addition, since certain types of problems, particularly genetic and developmental, are more common in children, they have resulted in subspecialties unique to pediatrics.

Increasingly, "obstetrics and gynecology" has been divided into the obstetrician who delivers babies and the gynecologist who deals with diseases of the female organs.

Psychiatry does not have formal subspecialties, but a variety of schools of psychotherapy exist—like Freudian and Jungian—which are somewhat similar to subspecialties in the other disciplines. Recently, obesity, alcoholism, and other specific problems have started to become subjects for separate disciplines within psychiatry.

The different kinds of doctors listed in this chapter provide their services under various arrangements. Sometimes, they practice alone, sometimes in groups, often under different financial conditions. You should know the strengths and weaknesses of each. By combining the right doctor with your medical and financial needs, you have a better chance of good medical care.

SOLO PRACTICE

The solo practitioner is just that—a physician without partners or organizational affiliation. The solo practitioner may be a general practitioner, a specialist, or a subspecialist in any of the medical disciplines. The solo practitioner generally works from an office which may or may not be near a hospital. With a solo practitioner, each time you are sick you will probably be seen by the same person. In small communities and rural areas, a solo practitioner may be the only source of medical care.

In recent years, busy solo practitioners have sometimes employed "physician's assistants" to enable them to care for a larger number of patients. Use of the "physician's assistant" is still undergoing evaluation, but early experience indicates that these health professionals, who are not themselves doctors, may provide excellent care in many areas of medicine.

It is rumored that, in the old days, a doctor was always available. One doubts that this was ever true; at any rate, it is not true now. The typical solo practitioner spends several weeks of the year on vacation or attending medical meetings. The doctor goes to concerts and parties like everybody else. A weekend may be spent at a cabin in the mountains. Obviously, such diversions are important for the mental health of the physician. On the other hand, these factors mean that you will not always see the same physician, even if your doctor is a solo practitioner. Upon reaching your doctor's answering service, you may be referred to another physician who is "on call."

GROUP PRACTICE

The medical group or "group practice" came into being some years ago as an answer to some of the problems of single practice. The sharing of night and weekend coverage, the lowering of office cost by shared expense, the availability of consultation, and a more medically stimulating environment for the physician all contributed to the increase in group practices. Group practices come in all sizes and varieties. The smallest group practice is the partnership; there may be two partners, or more. The partners may be incorporated into a "medical corporation."

The larger groups include hundreds of physicians. The group practice may include only general practitioners or only specialists in a particular area such as internal medicine. Other groups include a variety of medical specialties. Group practice has a number of advantages. You may be able to obtain a variety of medical services at a single location; the physicians will frequently have an organized education program which will assist in keeping them up-to-date; and there is likely to be a reliable on-call system.

On the other hand, a medical group is frequently more expensive than the solo practitioner, because members tend to refer you to other doctors. You may or may not see the same physician in the medical group at each visit, depending upon the design of the practice. Also, some patients have felt that relationships are more impersonal in these larger medical practices.

PAYING THE BILL

The quality of medical care is *not* determined by the method of payment; nevertheless, there are psychological factors in payment arrangements which every patient should understand.

Fee-for-service is an awkward term which describes the usual method of paying the doctor in the United States. A service is performed, and payment is given for that service. The more services provided, the greater the patient's bill. The more services provided, the greater the physician's income. In a country where nearly everyone is paid by salary, the existence of piece-work payment in medicine has raised criticism.

When payment is determined by the number of services, there is a financial incentive to increase the number of services provided and/or to up-grade their level. In the business sense, "customer satisfaction" becomes important to the physician. A good "bedside manner" may be developed and extra services may be provided in response to special problems. Since considerable effort is expended in maintaining the relationship with the patient, respect of physicians by patients tends to be greatest in areas where physicians are paid for each service.

On the other hand, some problems have been attributed to this payment system. It has been charged that patients have been seen too frequently, given too many medications, given too many shots, had too many diagnostic procedures performed, and undergone too much surgery as a result of this financial incentive. Studies have suggested that the physician in the fee-for-service setting provides many more services than physicians paid by salary. Controversy remains as to whether these additional services represent better care, or simply greater expense.

In *prepaid* practice, a group of physicians offers to the patient a plan which looks like an insurance policy; to the physician it represents a re-arrangement of the traditional incentives. The patient knows in advance the medical expenses for the year. A set monthly amount is paid regardless of whether the medical facility is used a great deal or isn't required at all. When the patient needs a doctor, little or no additional expense is involved. The physician is now given an incentive to *minimize* the number of services provided, since the amount of money to be earned is already determined.

Advocates of prepayment have argued that the physician has an incentive toward "preventive medicine" and is more likely to treat conditions early rather than to let them get out of hand. Close observers doubt that this is true. Little attention has been placed on preventive medicine by most prepaid group practices; indeed, sometimes the very opposite has been observed. However, prepaid group practices do decrease the overall cost of medical care. Usually, the saving is about 20 percent. Studies which compare the quality of medical care under the different payment conditions have not shown a difference; thus, the average patient in the prepaid medical plan saves money and avoids the nuisance of excessive medical procedures with no apparent decrease in the quality of the health care.

On the negative side, many patients are not happy with prepaid group practices. The most common complaints are that lines are too long, the physician too impersonal, and that they "feel like a number." These systems have been burdened by the few patients that over-use the system. In many plans, 20% of the patients use 80% of the services. The excessive services received by these few people increase the payments for the rest. The pre-paid group practice has a less direct stake in patient satisfaction than does the fee-for-service physician. As noted, the physician is now given the incentive to minimize the number of services provided since the amount of money is already determined. The dedication of most physicians counteracts these financial forces; with many doctors, these factors are unimportant. Still, you as the patient should be aware of the biases inherent in the care you receive.

WHICH DOCTOR IS RIGHT FOR YOU?

Given the choice of many kinds of physicians, medical practices, and payment schedules, which doctor is right for *you*? Medically, seeing different physicians every time seems to work out about as well as seeing the same physician consistently, if the medical record is of good quality or if the problems are acute. However, many patients and physicians feel that the dignity and depth of the relationship is impaired if frequent doctor changes are made.

Here are some things to remember when choosing a physician:

Usually, the *type* of physician is not as important as the individual physician. You can go to a general practitioner, a family doctor, a pediatrician, an internist, or a subspecialty internist for your primary care. Sometimes, women may use a gynecologist as their primary physician and have a Pap smear, breast examination, and blood pressure check during routine visits.

If you have a defined special problem, then a subspecialist in that area may be the best physician for you. The majority of your care can be provided and referral elsewhere arranged when it is needed.

You may want everyone in your family to see the same physician. This avoids the inconvenience of having several different doctors. More important, the physician who sees the entire family is better able to understand individual problems.

Rely upon your friends' experiences with their doctors. Question them closely about office practices. When the name of a physician is needed and you have not been able to obtain reliable information elsewhere, call your county medical society. They will have a list of physicians in the area who will accept new patients. Note that the medical society is providing information—not making recommendations; any member of the local society who is available may be given to you as a name. If you live near a medical school, you can find a doctor by getting the names of their clinical faculty.

When choosing a doctor, do not pay attention to the social status of the office address, the depth of the carpet, the clothing of the staff, or the hair style of the physician. Also, don't worry particularly about the length of the wait. The practice of medicine requires that the physician's working day be busy, that some problems require more time than others, and that emergencies may arise in the middle of the day. Hence, delays occur in the best organized practices, particularly with the most conscientious physicians. Take something useful to do to the doctor's office; don't count on the office magazines. The central question is this: Is this physician acting in the best interests of each patient he or she is seeing? You may need this special attention later.

HOW TO DETECT POOR MEDICAL SERVICE

There are some tip-offs to poor medical service. If you are taking three or more medicines of different types daily, you are usually getting poor advice unless you have a serious medical problem. If nearly every visit to the physician results in an injection, be a little suspicious. Be wary when any service costing a significant amount of money is promoted enthusiastically even though you were not aware of the need. If your questions go unanswered or if the physician fails to perform any physical examination at all, it's time to worry.

Under each of the medical problems in Section II, we have let you know what to expect at the doctor's office. If the physician does not perform these actions, there is cause for some questioning. Expectations indicated in this book are conservative and should be met in large part by most good physicians.

In the United States, free choice of physicians is available. For the "free market" to work effectively, you must be willing to "vote with your feet." In other words, if you cannot communicate effectively with your physician, seek another physician. If your questions are not adequately answered, go somewhere else. If practice does not live up to your expectations and to the guidelines of this book, select another physician.

But remember, your physician is human too. The physician is faced with a continual parade of diseases which cannot be changed by treatment, residing in the bodies of patients who demand treatment. Don't use the physician for trivial problems. Don't work to slowly erode medical ethics by requests for slightly misleading insurance claims, exaggerated disability statements, and repeated prescriptions for pain medication. The high ethical standards of our profession continue to impress us; still, human is human, and sometimes problems begin with the unconscious manipulations of patients.

Support good medical practices and become a committed medical consumer. If you believe that women should be in medicine, don't avoid them when you seek your own personal care. If you would like to see more general physicians in this country, don't seek a specialist to direct your own care. If you like house-calls, revere and respect the physician who will make them. If you want physicians to settle in your geographical area, patronize the physician closest to your home. If cost is important to you, comparison shop.

Using the guidelines presented in this chapter, you can arrange for the proper physician and payment system that will best fit your medical needs.

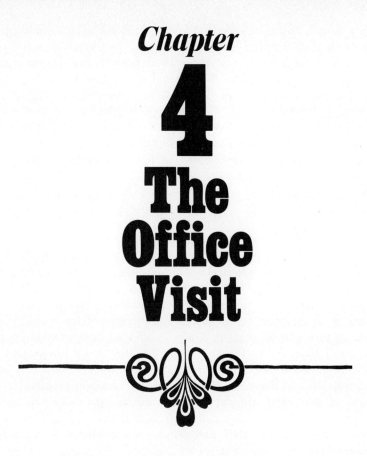

Chapter 4
The Office Visit

A visit to the doctor's office can often be a mysterious undertaking for many patients. This chapter will help you understand the general procedures a physician follows when you come to the office with a medical problem. In addition it will stress the importance of your active participation in these procedures and the advantages of strictly following your doctor's instructions.

THE MEDICAL HISTORY: TELLING IT LIKE IT IS

The "Medical History" is the most important communication between the patient and the physician. The ability to give a concise, organized description of your illness is essential to good care. The patient who rambles on about irrelevant details and doesn't mention real fears and problems is his or her own worst enemy. Inability to give a good medical history is expensive in terms of both your dollars and your health.

Most people do not realize that every physician uses a similar process to learn a patient's medical history. Obviously, the physician must organize information to be able to remember it accurately and reason correctly. Knowledge of the process can help you give accurate information to your doctor. The physician organizes information under five headings: the chief complaint, the present illness, the past medical history, the review of systems, and the social history. Physicians will not always request information in the same order, but the following definitions will help you recognize the purposes of the medical interview in which you are participating.

THE CHIEF COMPLAINT

Following the initial greeting, the "chief complaint" is usually the first information sought by the physician. This question may take several forms: "What bothers you the most?", "What brings you here today?" "What's the trouble?", or "What is your biggest problem?" The purpose of such questions is to establish the priorities for the rest of the medical history process. Be sure you get it right. Know in advance how to state your chief complaint: "I have a sore throat." "I have a pain in my lower right side." Any of the problems listed in the second section of this book may be your chief complaint, and there are hundreds of less common problems.

Think of the "chief complaint" as the *title* for the story you are about to tell the doctor. Do not give details of your illness at this time. Instead, title your illness appropriately and provide the doctor with a framework for understanding your problem.

Sometimes, you may go to the physician with more than one problem. You may not be sure whether the problems are related or not. Identify this situation for the doctor. "I seem to have three problems: sore throat, skin rash, and cloudy urine." The physician may then investigate each of these areas.

Tell it like it is. If you have a sexual problem, do not say that your chief complaint is that you're "tired and run down." If you are afraid that you have cancer, do not say that you came for a "checkup." If you mislead the physician because of embarrassment, the real reason for your visit may never be determined. You will compromise the physician's ability to be of assistance. An honest description is your best guarantee of having your problems attended correctly.

THE PRESENT ILLNESS

Next, your physician will want to hear the story behind the chief complaint. This section of the interview will be introduced by a question such as: "When did this problem begin?", "When were you last entirely well?", or "How long has this been going on?" The first fact which the physician wishes to establish is *how long* you have had the problem. Know the answer to this question in advance. "Yesterday." "On June 4th." "About the middle of May." If you are uncertain as to the date the problem began, state the uncertainty and tell what you can. "I am not sure when these problems began. I began to feel tired in the middle of February but the pain in the joints did not begin until the end of April." The physician can then determine the starting point for the illness.

After you define the starting point for the problem, the doctor will want to establish the sequence of events from that time until the present. Tell the story in the order it occurred. Do not use "flashbacks"; you will only confuse yourself and your physician. Do not attempt to tell everything you can remember about the illness, but highlight those events which seemed most important to you. Use short, concise sentences. Do not include irrelevant occurrences in your family or social situation. Your cause is not aided by reference to the relatives who were visiting you at the time, the purchases you made at the shopping center, or the state of international affairs. If you confuse your story, the chances for a successful solution to your problems are decreased.

As you recount the sequence of the problem, sketch the highlights as you perceive them:

> *I was well until I developed a sore throat four weeks ago. I had fever and some swollen glands in my neck. This lasted about a week and then I felt better although still tired. One week ago the fever returned. I began to have pains in my joints, beginning with the right knee. The joint pain moved around from one joint to another and I had pain in shoulders, elbows, knees and ankles. Over the last three days I have had a red rash over much of my body. I have not taken any medications except aspirin, which helps a little.*

The physician may interrupt the story to ask specific questions. At the end of the story questions may be asked about problems which you have not mentioned. By making your account well organized and allowing the physician to request additional information, you provide information in the most effective way.

If you have several problems to recount, the story of each may be told separately, or they may be intertwined in a single narrative. The physician may provide guidance to the most appropriate procedure in the individual case.

Supporting information may be extremely important. Know which medications you have taken before and during the course of the present illness. If necessary, bring the medication bottles to the physician. If you are pregnant or could be pregnant, tell the physician. If x-rays or laboratory tests have been performed during the course of the illness, attempt to make these materials or a report of the results available to the physician. If you are allergic to any drugs, mention these. If other physicians have been consulted, bring those medical records with you. Attempt to be a careful observer of your own illness. Your observations, if carefully made and recounted, are more valuable than any other source of information.

THE PAST MEDICAL HISTORY

After hearing your chief complaint and a history of your medical problem, your physician will want to know more background information about your general health. At this point, information which did not appear important earlier may become so. The physician will ask specific questions and will be assisted by direct, reasonably brief answers. You will be asked about your general health, hospitalizations, operative procedures, allergies, and medications. The physician may be interested in childhood illnesses as well as those occurring during adult life. (These should be recorded in Section III.)

The subjects most frequently misreported are allergies and medications. If you report a drug allergy, describe the specific reaction which you experienced. Many drug side effects (such as nausea, vomiting, or ringing in the ears) are *not* allergic in origin. Physicians are rightfully wary of prescribing drugs to which an allergy has been reported. If you report an allergy to a drug to which you are not allergic, you may deprive yourself of a useful method of treatment. When reporting medications, be complete. Birth control pills, vitamins, aspirin, and laxatives are medications. Frequently, the taking of these drugs is not reported. On occasion, each of these may be important in diagnosis or treatment of your medical problem.

THE REVIEW OF SYSTEMS

Next, your physician will usually review symptoms related to the different body systems from head to toe. There are standard questions for each system. Your physician may begin with questions about the skin, then ask about the head, eyes, ears, nose and throat, then begin to move down the body. Questions about the lymph glands, the lungs, and the heart are followed by questions about the stomach, intestines, and urinary system. Finally there will be questions asked about muscles, bones, and the nervous systems. In this questioning, the physician is looking for information which may have been missed previously, and for additional factors which may influence the choice of therapy. A very detailed "review of systems" will only be taken when you are having a complete health examination.

THE SOCIAL HISTORY

Finally, questions relating to the "social history" are addressed. Here, the physician may wish to know about your job, family, and interpersonal stresses. Questions may concern smoking, drinking, use of drugs, and sexual activity. Exposures to chemical or toxic substances may be sought. Questions are sometimes intensely personal. However, the answers can be of the utmost importance in determining your illness and how it can best be treated. Again, a detailed social history should be expected only in a complete health examination.

The physician has three major sources of information: the medical history, the physical examination, and laboratory tests. Depending on the illnesses, any one of the three may be the most important. The medical history is the only source of information which is directly controlled by the patient. It is frequently termed "subjective" by physicians because the information cannot be directly verified. To the extent that you provide your physician with clear, accurate data, you increase the probability of an accurate diagnosis and successful treatment of your problem.

LEARN TO OBSERVE YOURSELF

The careful physical examination requires skill and experience. Some important observations can be made at home and if you can report accurate information on these points you can further help your doctor.

Temperature: Don't say "fever" or "running a temperature" or "burning up." Own a thermometer, read the instructions, practice shaking the thermometer down, and be able to report the exact temperature. If you have a small child, own a rectal thermometer and know how to use it.

Pulse: If the problem involves a rapid or forceful heartbeat, know exactly how fast. Feel a pulse in the arm or throat, or put an ear to the chest. Count the exact number of beats in an exact minute, or have someone do this for you. If you think that there is a problem with the pulse, check whether the beat is regular or irregular. Is the heart "skipping a beat," "turning flip-flops," "missing every other beat," or completely irregular? Often a pulse irregularity is gone by the time you reach the doctor. If you can describe it accurately, your doctor may be able to understand what happened. For more information, refer to Palpitations, Problem 53.

Breast: The mammary tissue is normally a bit lumpy. Adult women should carefully examine their breasts every few months in order to detect changes. Do not press the breast tissue between the fingers, but press it against the chest wall. Try several positions—lying, sitting and with the arm on that side raised over the head. Look particularly for differences between the two breasts. If you note a suspicious lump, see the doctor immediately. Many women delay out of fear. Please don't. Very few lumps are actually cancer, but if the lump *is* malignant it is important that it be removed early. Often the patient can feel a lump which the doctor misses; help the doctor locate the problem area. Detailed instructions for a self-examination can be found in "For Women Only."

Weight: Changes in weight are frequently very important. Know what your normal weight is. If the weight changes, know by how much, and over what period it changed.

Other Findings: Know your body. When something changes, report it accurately. A change in skin color, a lymph gland on the back of the neck, an increase in swelling in the legs, and many other new events are easily observed. Just as important, knowledge of your body will help you avoid reporting silly things. The "Adam's apple" is not a tumor, "knobs" on the lower ribs or pelvis are usually normal, the vertebrae at the lower neck normally sticks out like that, and there is a normal bump at the back of the head—the "knowledge bump." We have seen patients reporting each of these as emergencies.

LISTEN: FOLLOW YOUR DOCTOR'S INSTRUCTIONS

If you are a typical patient, you carry out less than one-half of the instructions given to you by your physician. Think back to your last encounter with your physician. After you started to feel better, did you discontinue the medication prematurely? Did you have pills left over from your last prescription? Did you honestly adhere to diet recommendations? Did you restrict or increase your activity as instructed? Did you take medication irregularly, or exactly as prescribed? When a new illness occurred in your family, did you use medication "left over" from a previous encounter? If you did none of these things, you are a remarkable patient.

Let's look at the consequences of not following instructions:

First, there is the obvious waste of your time and your money. You are seeking expensive advice. As indicated in this book, there are many occasions when you do not require such advice. However, after you seek advice, it is ridiculous not to obtain the benefits. After you have arranged transportation to your doctor's office, waited until you could be seen, spent time with a trained professional, proceeded to a pharmacy, purchased medication, and finally returned home, you have invested a considerable amount of time and effort. Don't waste it by not following instructions.

Second, there are serious medical consequences if you don't follow instructions. The disease may persist; it may come back; you may have complications, side-effects, or drug interactions. The most frequent of these is that your problem may persist. For example, if you have an ulcer, the pain will usually respond within a few days to appropriate treatment. However, the ulcer crater, often large enough to stick your thumb into, has barely begun to heal. If treatment is not continued throughout a period of about six weeks, complete healing of the ulcer crater may not occur and the symptoms of the persisting condition may recur as soon as treatment is discontinued.

With urinary tract infection, the symptoms of urinary burning, lower abdominal pain, and frequent urination usually disappear in the first forty-eight hours of treatment. However, the bacteria which are responsible for the condition may not be totally destroyed for several more days. If antibiotic treatment is not continued until the condition is under control, the infection may come back, necessitating repeated medical attention. As another example, you may not realize that when you go to the physician for a sore throat, your physician is treating you mainly to prevent complications. Serious complications of strep throat include damage to the heart (acute rheumatic fever) and to the kidneys. These complications are unusual if ten days of antibiotic therapy is taken. However, you will feel well after forty-eight hours and may neglect further therapy. This is a major reason that long-acting penicillin shots may be prescribed for strep throats, since the physician is certain by giving you an injection that you will receive all the medication. In every scientific study, shots have proved superior to medication taken by mouth in preventing complications. Oral medication is not inferior, but patients are not reliable in taking it.

Sometimes patients take *too much* medication. Many operate on the theory that if a little bit is good, a lot is better. All drugs are alien to the body and basically must be considered to be "poisons." When used in excess of recommended dosage, you may encounter increased side-effects, dependence, addiction, or even death. You are gambling with your life if you increase the dosage when you do not know if this is safe.

Finally, drug interactions may occur. If a patient fails to report what medication is being taken, the physician may prescribe a new drug which has unfortunate interactions with the original medication. This represents a breakdown in your communication with your physician.

Most important, the patient who disregards instructions contributes to the dissipation of trust between patient and physician. Frequently, the patient who most strongly maintains that the physician "never explains things" is the same patient who disregards instructions. Not following "doctor's orders" puts a fundamental dishonesty into the patient-physician relationship. Future events cannot be correctly interpreted by the physician without accurate historical information. As a result, you receive more shots and fewer medications by mouth, while frequent visits are ordered so that the physician can check up on you. More blood tests are ordered to measure the actual blood levels of drugs you are supposed to be taking. Directness and honesty in the communication between doctor and patient are essential.

UNDERSTAND AND ADHERE TO YOUR DOCTOR'S PROGRAM

First, insist on understanding the importance of the medication and the instructions. Secondly, consider whether following the instructions poses any special problems. Third, adhere to the agreed program. Fourth, if medication remains after the course of therapy, destroy it.

You must understand the instructions given to you. If you are confused, ask questions: "Could you go over that again?" "I don't understand what this medication is for." "Do I really have to be treated in the hospital?" "How much will this cost?" "Are there any risks to this drug?" Ask your doctor to write out the instructions. Understand the importance of each drug or treatment. In some instances it does not matter if you take the medicine regularly; in these circumstances the drug gives only symptomatic relief and should be discontinued as soon as possible. Be sure that you understand whether it is or is not necessary to continue the medication when you feel well.

Consider the entire prescribed program. You may have difficulties not known to your physician. Perhaps you have trouble taking a medication at work. Perhaps you anticipate trouble with a prescribed diet. Perhaps reasons unknown to your physician prevent your undertaking the recommended activity. If more than one medication has been prescribed initially, it may be more desirable for you to take them all at once. When such questions arise, ask in advance. Frequently, if you raise these questions with your physician, your treatment program can be modified so that you can feel more comfortable. The keynote is honesty. Don't say that you will do something which you know you will not do. Express your worries.

After an agreed program has been prescribed, follow it closely. If you notice possible side-effects from the program, call the physician and inquire. If side-effects are serious, return for examination. Make a chart of the days of the week, and the times when medications are to be taken. Note on the chart when you take the medicines. Don't look on this as an insult to your intelligence; this practice is universally used in hospitals by trained personnel to insure that medication schedules are maintained accurately. At home, you and your family are the custodians of your health. Do not take this task more lightly than it is taken by professionals.

When pills remain at the end of a course of therapy, flush them down the toilet. There are multiple hazards with a medicine chest containing old prescription medicines. Every year, children and adults die from taking left-over drugs. Children take birth control pills, adults brush their teeth with steroid creams, and the wrong medication is taken because another bottle was thought to be in hand. If you give your leftover tetracycline to your children with their next cold, you are probably not aware that you may cause mottling of their teeth. If the same tetracycline becomes outdated and is subsequently used, you are probably not aware that dangerous liver damage may result. When a new illness occurs, the situation is confused if you have already taken left-over medications. Sometimes it will be impossible to make an accurate identification of a bacteria by culture or the clinical picture of the disease may be distorted.

The doctor-patient encounter is your most reliable protection against *serious* illness. Value the opportunity for such attention, utilize it selectively, and follow to the maximum extent possible the instructions you are given.

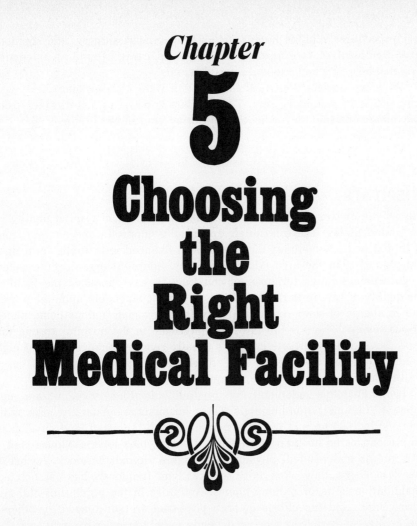

Chapter

5

Choosing the Right Medical Facility

A wide variety of medical facilities are available to prospective patients—hospitals, emergency rooms, convalescent homes, and clinics. There are choices for most tastes and for the satisfaction of most individuals. It's important to know the facilities in your area and to make your choices before you need the services.

To select the best facilities, you will need to understand the terms "primary," "secondary," and "tertiary" care. *Primary* medical care is provided by a physician at the office or at an emergency room or clinic. It is care which may be obtained by a patient without the referral of another physician. It is often called "ambulatory care" or "out-patient care." *Secondary* care is that afforded by the typical community hospital and the physicians involved may be specialists or subspecialists. As a rule, access to this care requires the referral of a physician. Much secondary care is "in-patient" or hospital care. *Tertiary* care includes special and extraordi-

nary procedures such as kidney dialysis, open-heart surgery, and sophisticated treatment of rare diseases. This type of care is found at university
affiliated hospitals and regional referral centers.

When you select a medical facility, you want close primary care with
good access to secondary care. Tertiary care is often a great distance from
your home, and may never be needed during your entire lifetime.

HOSPITALS

The *private* or *community hospital* is the most common hospital facility in
the United States. These hospitals are usually nonprofit, and contain from
50 to 400 beds. Sometimes they have been financed with funds from doctors practicing in the area. More frequently, nonprofit organizations aided
by government funds for hospital construction have financed the facility.
The quality of care in these institutions is largely dependent upon the physician in charge of your case. Relatively few physician actions come under
serious review. There is not always a physician in the hospital around the
clock. Nevertheless, private hospitals usually give personalized care of high
quality. The hospital is quiet and orderly. In the great majority of cases
facilities are adequate for the care required.

Public hospitals include city, county, public health service, military, and
Veterans Administration hospitals. These hospitals are generally large, with
from 500 to 1000 beds. They have permanent full-time staff, and physicians
are present in the hospital at all times. Usually, they have a "house staff,"
with interns and resident physicians available around the clock. As befits
their larger size, they offer more services, and frequently have associated
rehabilitation units or nursing homes. Activities in the public hospital are
more visible, and the efforts of each physician are scrutinized by others.
The quality of care you receive depends upon the overall quality of the
institution. The presence of interns and residents may pose some minor
inconveniences to you as a patient, however, their presence is an excellent
guarantee of good care. The physician-in-training has patient care as his or
her primary responsibility, and is not greatly involved with office practice
and administrative tasks.

Many public hospitals have the reputation for providing service to a
poorer economic class. Within the community, they are often perceived as
offering substandard service. Usually, these accusations are grossly unfair.
While not always quiet and orderly, and often not physically attractive,
these hospitals give dependable and excellent care. When available, they
should be seriously considered by individuals in all economic classes.

The *teaching hospital* is one associated with a medical school. Teaching
hospitals are large, with a range of from 300 to 2000 beds. These hospitals
always have interns and residents and additionally have medical students
on the hospital wards. They have superb technical resources, and it is here
that the most extraordinary events of medicine take place. Open-heart

surgery, transplantation of kidneys, elaborate nurseries for the newborn, support for management of rare blood diseases, and other marvels are all available here. Dozens of people may be concerned with the wellbeing of a particular patient. Crucial medical decisions are thoroughly discussed, presented at conferences, and reviewed by many personnel.

On the other hand, the quality of personal relationships at teaching hospitals is variable. Many patients feel that they are treated in an impersonal way, and that their laboratory tests receive more attention than their human and social problems. Since these institutions are on the frontier of medicine, there is a tendency to emphasize the new and elaborate procedures, when older and more modest ones might have served as well. With the inexperience of some members of the care team, there is a tendency to order more laboratory tests than would have been ordered for the same condition in a private hospital. The sick patient is sometimes confused by having to relate to a large number of doctors and students. Medical educators are concerned with such criticisms, and have moved to correct some of the problems. However, some excesses of technological medicine still occur in these institutions.

KNOW WHEN TO USE THE HOSPITAL

The hospital is expensive. It is not home or hotel. It saves lives and it takes them. It must be used and it must be avoided. To manage these contradictions, the need for hospitalization for you or your family must be carefully considered in each instance.

Don't use the hospital if services can be performed outside the hospital. The acute general hospital does acute general medicine well; it does not do other functions well.

Don't use the hospital for a rest; it is not a good place to rest. It is busy, noisy, unfamiliar, and populated with strange roommates. Its nights are punctuated with interruptions, and it has an unusual time schedule. It has many employees, a few of whom are less thoughtful than others.

Don't use the hospital for the "convenience" of having a number of tests done in a few days. It does not provide tests in the most efficient manner; indeed, most laboratories and x-ray facilities are not open on the weekend, and special procedures may require several days just to be scheduled.

Many have urged that we have a system of "hoptels," which provide lodging at minimal cost, allow for efficient test performance, and are appropriate for periods of rest and minimal activity. A number of experiments along these lines are underway. Until more appropriate facilities are available, however, use the acute hospital with great reluctance.

A century ago, the Hungarian physician, Inaz Philipp Semmelweiss (1818–1865), noted that both infants and mothers delivering at home fared better than those in the hospital and that the existence of often fatal "childbed fever" was one of the risks of the hospital. This problem, due to poor hygiene in the delivery rooms, has long since been corrected. But in our present age, new evidence suggests that for many conditions home treatment may work better than treatment in the hospital. For example, treatment for minor heart attacks at home has been reported as possibly better than treatment in a hospital. It is apparent to most hospital visitors that the crisis atmosphere of the acute hospital does not promote the calmest state of mind for the patient. Many therapeutic features of the home cannot be duplicated in the hospital.

EMERGENCY ROOMS

The emergency room has become the "physician" for many patients. Patients who cannot find a physician at night, or who don't know where else to go are coming to emergency rooms with increased frequency. The typical emergency room is now filled with nonemergency cases. Trivial illnesses which could have been treated with the aid of this book, routine problems more easily and economically handled in a physician's office, specialized problems which should have been seen at a time when the hospital facilities were fully available, and true emergencies are all mixed together. Even though the emergency room is not designed for the purpose it now serves, it does a surprisingly good job of delivering adequate care.

However, there are major disadvantages to an emergency room as the sole medical contact. Emergency rooms make little or no provision for continued care. In the emergency room you will usually be seen by different physicians. The emergency room physician will attend to the chief problem reported by the patient but seldom has sufficient time to complete a full examination or to deal with underlying problems. While simple x-ray facilities are available, procedures such as gallbladder studies and upper G.I. series are arranged with difficulty. Thus, evaluation of a complicated problem is not well handled by the emergency room. When a true emergency occurs, patients with less urgent problems are shunted to the end of the line. You cannot estimate with any certainty how long it will take you to be seen in an emergency room. Emergency room fees, because they support equipment required to handle true emergencies, are higher than those of standard office visits. Emergency room services are not always covered by medical insurance, even when the policy states that the costs of emergency care are included. With many policies, the nature of the illness governs whether or not it is covered. You may end up paying a large bill if you go to the emergency room with a sore throat.

The smoothly functioning emergency room is a dramatic place and provides one of the finest examples of a service profession at work. Using the procedures outlined in this book, you can use this valuable resource appropriately.

Recently a number of facilities specially designed for surgery which requires only a short stay (overnight at the most) have appeared. Obviously such surgery is minor and the patient must basically be in good health. Since such centers are able to avoid some of the overhead of a hospital, they often can charge you less for the use of their facilities. But, since they do not have the capability to handle difficult cases or complications, you should use them only when the procedure is truly minor.

CONVALESCENT FACILITIES

Nursing homes and various types of rehabilitation facilities provide for the patient who does not require more expensive care but cannot be adequately managed at home. These facilities range from abysmal to superb. In the best circumstances, with dedicated nursing and regular physician attendance, a comfortable and homelike situation for the patient can accelerate the healing process. In other cases, disinterest, inadequate facilities, and minimal care are the rule. Before suggesting or accepting referral to a nursing home facility, visit the facility or have a friend or relative visit it for you. In the convalescent setting, your comfort with the arrangements is essential.

FREE CLINICS

In many areas of the country, "free clinics" have developed.

In some cases, they have appeared because the general medical care in the community has been poor. In others, clinics have developed to deal with undesired pregnancies, drug use, and venereal disease. These clinics are high in idealism and usually short in money. Sympathetic care from sensitive individuals is the rule. Facilities will be limited, but considerable thought will have been given to those services included, so that relatively little is lost.

These clinics provide care for many who would not find it available elsewhere. However, the financial instability and the political ferment of many free clinics make their continued existence uncertain; these clinics come into and go out of existence with regularity. Free clinics do not present any challenge to organized medicine but serve to remind it of its inequities. In most cases, they deserve much broader community support than they receive.

It will be worth your time to investigate the various medical facilities in your area. If you can, visit them and ask questions. "Is there emergency care?" "Is there always a doctor on duty?" "What are your payment arrangements?" Then choose the facilities that will best meet your needs.

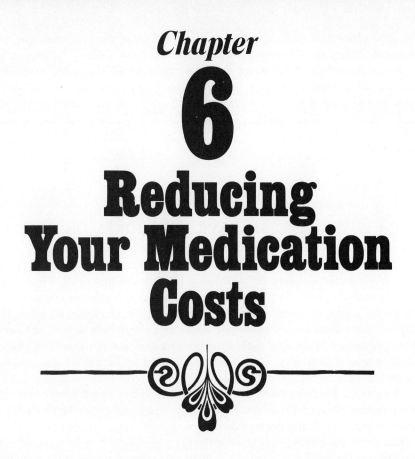

Chapter

6

Reducing Your Medication Costs

Legal drugs are a multibillion dollar industry. Your contribution to this industry is largely voluntary. The size of the contribution is determined by your illness, your physician, your pharmacy, and yourself.

Drugs are life-saving, dangerous, curative, painful, pain-relieving, and easy to misuse. Also, they are basically poisons. Drugs interact with other drugs causing hazardous chemical reactions. They have direct toxic reactions on the stomach lining and elsewhere in the body. They cause allergic rashes and shock. They are foreign chemicals with severe toxic effects when taken in excess. Under some circumstances they probably cause cancers, and some drugs decrease the ability of the body to fight infections.

If you do *not* receive a prescription or a sample package of medication from your physician, consider this good news rather than rejection. Prefer to take the fewest possible drugs for the shortest possible time. When drugs are prescribed, take them regularly and as directed, but expect that your medication program will be reviewed, thoroughly, every time you see your doctor.

Most drugs are given as "symptomatic medications," that is, they do not cure your problem, but attempt only to give some relief for the symptoms of that problem. If you report a new minor symptom every time you see your physician, and urgently request relief from the symptom, you will probably be given additional medications. You are unlikely to feel much better as the result of the extra medications, and you are nearly certain to function at a lower level as a human being. Unless you have a serious illness, you seldom should be taking more than one or two medications at a time. Perceptive observers have argued that the present practice of using drugs to control symptoms is only a temporary phase in the history of medicine.

YOUR PHYSICIAN CAN SAVE YOU MONEY ON DRUGS

Your physician plays a major role in the cost of drugs by choosing the drugs to be prescribed. For example, if you have an infection due to bacteria, you may be given tetracycline or erythromycin. Tetracycline costs about three cents a capsule, while erythromycin costs about twenty-five cents. If you are given a steroid prescription for asthma, at the physician's option this may be prednisone at two cents per tablet or methylprednisolone at twenty cents per tablet. Medically, such drug choices are between agents of similar effectiveness. If your physician prescribes a drug by its trade name, in most states the pharmacist must fill the prescription with that particular brand-name product. The brand-name product frequently has a cost many times that of its "generic" equivalent. Does your physician know the relative cost of alternative drugs? Many doctors do not.

The drug-prescribing habits of different physicians can be divided into two groups: the "additive" and the "substitutive" prescribers. With an "additive" physician, each visit you receive a medication *in addition* to those which you already have. With a "substitutive" prescribing physician, the medication you were previously taking is discontinued and a new medicine is *substituted*. Usually, the "substitutive" practice is advantageous to your health as well as your pocketbook.

Most of the time, medication can be taken orally. The common reason for requiring medication by injection is the physician's uncertainty that you will take the medication as prescribed; by injecting it, the medication certainly has been taken. As a thoughtful and reliable patient, however, you can assure your physician of compliance with an oral regimen. Taking medication orally is less painful, less likely to result in an allergic reaction, and far less expensive. There are exceptions, but you should seek oral medication when possible.

If it is clear that you must take a medication for a prolonged period, ask the physician to allow refills on the prescription. With many drugs it is not necessary to be charged an additional physician visit just to get a prescription written. Under other circumstances, the physician may wish to examine you before deciding whether the drug can be safely continued or is still required. Ask your physician if refills on the prescription are permitted.

The careful physician will ensure that you fully understand each drug that you are taking, the reasons you are taking it, the side effects which may possibly arise, and the expected length of time that you will be taking the medication. A medication schedule will be arranged during the day so that it is convenient as well as medically effective. If the program is confusing, ask for written instructions. It is crucial that you understand the why and how of your drug therapy. Do not leave the physician's office for the pharmacy without understanding your medications.

REDUCING COSTS AT THE PHARMACY

The pharmacy is another crucial factor in your drug expenses. For the most part, the pharmacist no longer weighs and measures individual chemical formulations. Much of the activity in the pharmacy consists of relabeling and dispensing manufactured medication. Medication is thus usually identical at different pharmacies; you should choose the least expensive and the most convenient. Comparison shop. Often discount stores will offer the same medication at significantly lower prices. If a considerable sum of money is involved, you should compare prices by telephone before purchase. If a pharmacy won't give you price information over the phone, don't go to it.

Unfortunately, even though your physician writes a prescription by "generic" name rather than brand name, the pharmacist is not required to give you the cheapest of the equivalent alternatives. Often, the pharmacy will stock only one manufacturer's formulation of each drug. Thus, even though your physician has been careful to allow the pharmacist to substitute a less expensive preparation, the pharmacist may not do so because only a more expensive alternative is in stock. There is no way to detect this problem except to get direct price quotes from different pharmacies.

The majority of pharmacies charge a percentage markup. Their pricing is determined by the wholesale price, multiplied by a fixed profit figure. A sliding scale may be used, but profit is largest on the largest sales. Other pharmacies work on a specific charge per prescription. These pharmacies take the wholesale price and add a constant fee. With a small drug bill, you will be better with the percentage mark-up formulas. If you are buying a significant quantity of expensive medication, application of the one-time fixed charge may be less costly. Knowledge of these problems and aggressive comparison shopping is essential for the consumer to control costs.

ULTIMATELY, YOU CONTROL YOUR DRUG COSTS

You are the ultimate determinant of your drug cost. In this age, visits to the physician are frequently requests for medication. If your satisfaction with the physician depends on whether or not you are given medication, you are applying pressure against your own best interest. If you go to a physician because of a cold and request a "shot of penicillin," you are asking for poor medical practice. Penicillin should infrequently be given by injection, and it should not be given for uncomplicated colds. Your physician knows this but may give in to your pressure.

The most frequently prescribed medications in the United States, making up the bulk of drug cost, are *not* scientifically important medications. Instead, they are tranquilizers, minor pain relievers, and sedatives. These prescribing patterns arose, in large part, because of ill-advised consumer demand. You can decrease the cost of medications by using some of the techniques above; you can eliminate them almost completely by decreasing your pressure to receive and utilize medications which you do not require.

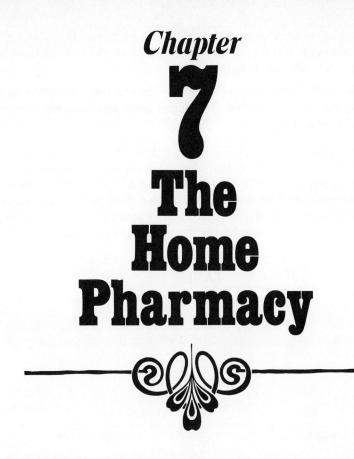

Chapter 7
The Home Pharmacy

To effectively treat the minor illnesses which appear from time to time in your family, you need to have some medications on hand, and to know where to obtain others as you need them. Your stock should include the most inexpensive and the most frequently needed medications. Even these will deteriorate with time and should be replaced at least every three years.

In this section we list the products for a typical home medical shelf and discuss the uses for each item. The guidelines for common medical problems in Section II of this book tell you when and why to use each medication. We provide some commentary upon dosage and side effects; since these are subject to changes, you should carefully read the instructions which come with the medication. Our comments will provide some critical perspective to the manufacturer's statements.

Reading the labels of compounds available at the supermarket can be a little frightening. It is in the manufacturer's interest to extoll the product's benefits while including strong warnings concerning its possible side effects in the small print. It is also in the manufacturer's interest to recommend the smallest dosage that is likely to have any effect. In short, you are exhorted to buy the drug but not to cause any trouble, especially legal trouble due to side effects. Be this as it may, you must accept certain truths about drugs:

- Used in effective dosages, all drugs have the potential for side effects. Some side effects, such as drowsiness, are impossible to avoid at effective dosages with many common drugs.

- Misuse of over-the-counter drugs can have serious consequences. Do not assume that a product is automatically safe because it does not require a prescription.

The rational approach to this dilemma is for you to learn something of the drugs which may be useful to you. This is the reason for this section.

There are many hundreds of over-the-counter medicines available at your supermarket or drugstore. For most purposes there are several medicines which are almost identical. This has posed a problem for us in the organization of this chapter: if we discuss drugs by chemical name the terms are

---

TABLE 1

◄ YOUR HOME PHARMACY ►

Items in bold print are basic requirements. Other preparations may find use in some households. Keep all medicines out of the reach of children.

Ailment	Medication
Allergy	Antihistamines Nose drops and sprays
Colds and Coughs	Cold tablets/cough syrups
Constipation	Milk of magnesia, bulk laxatives
Dental problems (preventive)	Sodium fluoride
Diarrhea	**KAOPECTATE, paregoric**
Eye irritations	Eye drops and artificial tears
Hemorrhoids	Hemorrhoid preparations
Pain and fever	**ASPIRIN, acetaminophen**
(in children)	† **LIQUID ACETAMINOPHEN, aspirin** rectal suppositories
Poisoning (to induce vomiting)	† **SYRUP OF IPECAC**
Fungus	Antifungal preparations
Sunburn (preventive)	Sunscreen agents
Sprains	**ELASTIC BANDAGES**
Stomach, upset	**ANTACID, nonabsorbable**
Wounds (minor)	**ADHESIVE TAPE, BANDAGES**
(antiseptic)	**HYDROGEN PEROXIDE, iodine**
(soaking agent)	**SODIUM BICARBONATE (baking soda)**

---

† Daggered items are for homes with small children.

long and confusing, while if we use the brand name we may appear to favor the product of a particular manufacturer when there are equally satisfactory alternatives. We have decided, instead, to give some clues to reading the list of ingredients on the package so that you can figure out what the drug is likely to do. We have included brand names in the index at the back of the book. We do not include all available drugs, but we do mention representative alternatives. The brand names listed in this chapter are vigorously marketed and should be available almost everywhere. They are *not necessarily* superior to alternatives, not listed, which contain similar formulas.

ALLERGY

Antihistamine Compounds: Allerest, Sinarest, Sinutab, Dristan

The many over-the-counter drugs designed for treatment of minor allergic symptoms are similar to the cold compounds described below, but less frequently contain pain and fever agents like aspirin or acetaminophen. Usually, these drug compounds contain an antihistamine and a decongestant agent, which can be identified from the label. If you tolerate one of these drugs well, and get good relief, it may be continued for several weeks (for example, through a hay fever season) without seeing a physician. The same sort of drug taken as nose drops or nasal spray should be used more sparingly and only for short periods, as detailed in Nose Drops and Sprays, below. You can purchase the ingredients of the compound separately and usually should.

Reading the labels: The decongestant is often phenylephrine, ephedrine, or phenylpropanolamine. If the compound name is not familiar, the suffix "ephrine" or "-edrine" will usually identify this component of the compound. The antihistamine is often chlorpheniramine (Chlor-trimeton) or pyrilamine. If not, the antihistamine is sometimes (but not always) identifiable on the label by the "-amine" suffix.

Dosage: As per product directions. Reduce dose if side effects are noted, or try another compound.

Side effects: These are usually minor and disappear after the drug is stopped or decreased in dose. Agitation and insomnia usually mean too much of the decongestant component. Drowsiness usually means too much antihistamine. If you can avoid the substance to which you are allergic, it is far superior to taking drugs which, to a certain degree, inevitably impair your functioning.

Nosedrops and Sprays: Afrin, Neo-Synephrine, Dristan, Sinarest, Contac

With a cold or allergy, the runny nose is often the worst symptom. Since this complaint is so common, it is big business. There are many remedies advertised for the purpose of decreasing nasal secretions. Many of these preparations are "topical," as with nose drops and sprays, and act directly on the inflamed tissue. There are some problems associated with use of these compounds.

The active ingredient in these compounds is a decongestant drug, usually ephedrine or phenylephrine. When applied, you can feel the membranes shrinking down and "drawing," and you note a decrease in the amount of secretion. In other words, the medication is effective, and can relieve symptoms.

The major drawback is that the relief is temporary. Usually the symptoms return in a couple of hours, and you repeat the dose. This is fine for a while. But, these drugs work by causing the muscle in the walls of the blood vessels to constrict, decreasing blood flow. After many applications, these small muscles become fatigued, and fail to respond. Finally, they are so fatigued that they relax entirely and the situation becomes worse than it was in the beginning. This is medically termed "rebound vasodilatation" and can occur if you use these drugs steadily for three days or more. Many patients interpret these increased symptoms as a need for more medication. Taking more only makes the problem worse and worse. Therefore, use nose drops or sprays only for a few days at a time. After several days rest, then they may be used again for a few days.

Dosage: These drugs are almost always used in the wrong way. If you can taste the drug you have applied it to the wrong area. If you don't bathe the swollen membranes on the side surface of the inner nose you won't get the desired effect. Apply small amounts to one nostril, then lie down on that side for a few minutes so that the medicine will bathe the membranes. Then apply the agent to the other side and lie down on that side. Treat four times a day if needed, but do not continue for more than three days without interrupting therapy.

Side effects: Rebound vasodilatation from prolonged use is the most common problem. If you apply these agents incorrectly and swallow a lot of the drug, you can get a rapid heart rate and an uneasy, agitated feeling. The drying effect can result in nosebleeds. Try to avoid the substances to which you are allergic rather than treating the consequences of exposure. Often simple measures like changing a furnace filter or using an air conditioner to filter the air will improve symptoms.

COLDS AND COUGHS

Cold Tablets: Coricidin, Dristan, Contac

Dozens of products are widely advertised as effective against the common cold, and the choice is confusing. Surprisingly, many give satisfactory symptomatic relief. While we do not feel that these compounds add much to standard treatment with aspirin and fluids, many patients feel otherwise, and we do not discourage their use for short periods.

The compounds usually have three basic ingredients. The most important is aspirin (or acetaminophen), which acts to reduce fever and pain. In addition, there is a decongestant drug which acts to shrink the swollen membranes and the small blood vessels, and an antihistamine which acts to block any allergy and to dry the mucus.

Reading the labels: The decongestant is often phenylephrine, ephedrine, or phenylpropanolamine. If the compound name is not familiar, the suffix "ephrine" or "edrine" will usually identify this component of the compound. The antihistamine is often chlorpheniramine (Chlor-trimeton) or pyrilamine. If not, the antihistamine is usually (but not always) identifiable on the label by the "-amine" suffix.

Occasionally, a "belladonna alkaloid" is added to these compounds to enhance other actions and reduce stomach spasms. In the small doses used there is little effect from these drugs, which are listed as "scopolamine," "belladonna," or something similar. Other ingredients which may be listed contribute little. Do not use products with caffeine if you have heart trouble or difficulty sleeping. Do not use products with phenacetin over a long period because kidney damage has been reported.

These products, then, contain the much promoted "combination of ingredients" approach. As a general rule, single drugs are preferable to combination; they allow you to be more selective in treatment of symptoms and you take fewer drugs. The ingredients in combination products are available alone and should be considered as alternatives. The major ingredient, aspirin, is discussed below. Pseudoephedrine is an excellent decongestant which is available without prescription in 30 mg tablets (the 60 mg tablets *do* require a prescription strangely enough; take two of the little ones if you are an adult). Chlorpheniramine, the antihistamine, is now available over-the-counter in the standard 4 milligram size. When possible, consider applying medicine directly to the affected area, as with nose drops or sprays for a runny nose.

Finally note that the commonly *prescribed* cold medicines (Sudafed, Actifed, Dimetapp) are really just more concentrated and expensive formulations of the same type of drugs. Is it worth a trip to the doctor just for that?

Dosage: Try the recommended dosage. If no effect is noted, you may increase the dosage by one-half. Do not exceed twice the recommended dosage. Remember that you are trying to find a compromise between desired effects and side effects. Increasing the dosage gives some chance of increased beneficial effects. It guarantees a greater probability of side effects.

Side effects: What puts one person to sleep will keep another awake. The most frequent side effects are drowsiness and agitation. The drowsiness usually comes from the antihistamine component and the insomnia or agitation from the decongestant component. You can try another compound which has less or none of the offending chemical, or you can reduce the dose. There are no frequent serious side effects; most dangerous is drowsiness if you intend to drive or operate machinery. Rarely, the "belladonna" component will cause dryness of mouth, blurring of vision, or inability to urinate. Aspirin's usual side effects may also be seen—upset stomach or ringing in the ears.

COUGH SYRUPS

This is a confusing area, with many products. To simplify a little, consider only two major categories of cough medication: "expectorants" and "cough suppressants." The expectorants are usually preferable, since they liquefy the secretions and allow the body's defenses to get rid of the bad material. Cough suppressants should be avoided if the cough is bringing up any material or if there is a lot of mucus. In the late stages of a cough, where it is dry and hacking, compounds containing a suppressant may be useful. We prefer compounds which do not contain an antihistamine since the drying effect on the mucus can hurt as much as help.

Reading the labels: Glyceryl guaiacolate, potassium iodide, chloroform, and several other frequently used chemicals cause an expectorant action. Cough suppressant action comes principally from narcotics, such as codeine. Over-the-counter cough suppressants cannot contain codeine. They often contain dextromethorphan hydrobromide, which is not a narcotic but is a close chemical relative. Many commercial mixtures contain a little of everything, and may have some of the ingredients of the cold compounds as well. We will discuss only glyceryl guaiacolate (Robitussin, 2/G) and dextromethorphan (Romilar) specifically; follow the label instructions for other agents.

Glyceryl Guaiacolate: Robitussin, 2/G

This cough medicine acts to draw more liquid into the mucus which triggers a cough, and thus to liquefy these mucus secretions so that they may be coughed free. The easier cough reduces irritation. With a dry hacking cough hanging on after a cold, the lubrication alone often soothes the inflamed area. The basic component in these medications, glyceryl guaiacolate, does not suppress the cough reflex, but encourages the natural defense mechanisms of the body. It is safe. It is not as powerful as the codeine-containing preparations, but for routine use we prefer it to prescription drugs. The two common brand-name products (Robitussin and 2/G) are medically equivalent but have a slightly different taste.

Reading the labels: These drugs are available also in combination with decongestants and actual cough suppressants; the decongestants may carry a "-PE" suffix for "phenylephrine" and the cough suppressants a "-DM" for "dextromethorphan."

Dosage: One or two teaspoonfuls three or four times daily for adults; half as much for children six to twelve; One-fourth teaspoon for children between one and six. Give your physician a call if you have a sick and coughing child less than a year old.

Side effects: No significant problems have been reported. If preparations containing other drugs are used, side effects from the other components of the combination may occur.

Dextromethorphan: Romilar

This drug "calms the cough center," which is to say that it makes the areas of the brain which control cough less sensitive to the stimuli which trigger coughs. No matter how much is used, it will seldom decrease cough by more than 50 percent. Thus, you cannot totally suppress a cough; this is probably not a bad thing since the cough is a protective reflex. This drug may be used with dry hacking coughs which are preventing sleep or work.

Dosage: Adults often require up to twice the recommended dosage to obtain any effect. Do not exceed twice the recommended dose. There is no further benefit and you may get into problems.

Side effects: Drowsiness is the only side effect reliably reported.

CONSTIPATION

We prefer a natural diet, with natural vegetable fiber residue, to the use of any laxative. But if you must use them, the most attractive alternatives are *psyllium* as a bulk laxative or *milk of magnesia* to hold water in the bowel and to soften the stool.

Bulk Laxatives: Metamucil, Effersylium

This substance can help both diarrhea and constipation. It draws water into the stool, forms a gel or thick solution, and thus provides bulk. It is a product refined from the psyllium seed. It is not absorbed by the digestive tract but only passes through; thus it is a natural product and one with essentially no contraindications and no side effects. With all this going for it, we must admit that it doesn't always work and that a similar effect can probably be obtained by eating enough celery. It has been recommended as a weight reduction aid when taken before meals because it induces a feeling of fullness which may reduce appetite, however, it doesn't seem very effective in this role.

Dosage: One teaspoonful, stirred in a glass of water, taken twice daily is a typical dose. A second glass of water or juice should also be taken. Psyllium is also available in more expensive, individual-dose packets, for times when you don't have a teaspoon. The effervescent versions mix a bit more rapidly and taste better to some.

Side effects: If taken with insufficient water, the gel which is formed could conceivably lodge in the esophagus (the tube which leads from mouth to stomach). Sufficient liquid will prevent this problem.

Milk of Magnesia

This home remedy has been on everybody's bathroom shelf since grandma's days. It has two actions: As a laxative it causes fluid to be retained within the bowel and in the feces; as an antacid it neutralizes the acid in the stomach. It is an effective antacid, but unfortunately, when taken in a sufficient dose to help an ulcer patient (see Antacids), it causes severe diarrhea. A single dose is relatively well tolerated, so a mild upset stomach may be treated with milk of magnesia.

As a laxative, the magnesium is the active ingredient. While it cannot be termed a "natural" laxative, it is mild and less subject to abuse than many alternatives.

Dosage: For the adult, 30 cc (two tablespoons) liquid may be taken at bedtime as a laxative or up to once daily, as required, to quiet stomach upset. It produces its laxative effect in approximately eight hours. If the stomach is not soothed, use *another* antacid more frequently. Children 6 to 12, one-half dose. Children 3 to 6, one-fourth dose. As with other antacids, two tablets are roughly equal to two tablespoons liquid in chemical content. However, the liquid is more effective as an antacid.

Side effects: This one is hard to get into trouble with, because you get diarrhea before any more serious effects. Too much magnesium is harmful to the body, but you won't get that much unless you go through a bottle a day. There is some salt present, so be careful if you are on a low-salt diet. Milk of magnesia is a "nonabsorbable" antacid, so it does not greatly affect the acidity of the body. However, it should *never* be used by persons with kidney disease.

DENTAL CARE

Take care of your teeth; they chew for you. There is good evidence that preventive measures can save teeth. By all means brush as recommended and use dental floss to clean the difficult areas between the teeth. Many doctors feel that flossing is the most important preventive for adult tooth decay. Also, make sure that children have an adequate fluoride intake each day.

Sodium Fluoride

If your water supply is fluoridated, your fluoride intake is adequate and you do not need to supplement. You must know if your water is fluoridated or not. If it is not, it is important for children's teeth that you supplement their diet with fluoride. There remains argument as to whether fluoride continues to be required after the teeth have been formed, but all authorities agree that fluoride is needed through age ten. To be sure, you may wish to continue it for several years longer, until all the molars are in. Adults probably do not require dietary fluoride, although the painting of teeth with fluoride paste by the dentist is still felt helpful, as is stannous fluoride toothpaste.

Dosage: Fortunately, it is relatively easy to supplement with fluoride when the water supply is not treated. Get a big bottle of fluoride tablets in a soluble form. Most tablets are 2.2 milligrams and contain 1 mgm of fluoride; the rest is a soluble sugar. A child under the age of three needs about ½ milligram per day, and a child between three and ten needs a full milligram, or one tablet. The tablets may be chewed or swallowed. They may also be taken in milk; they do not alter the taste. For example, if you have two children drinking milk, and a half-gallon lasts two days in your home, you need only place four tablets into the milk when you first open it, and they will dissolve and give the proper dose. In states where fluoride is available only by prescription, request a prescription from your doctor or dentist on a routine visit.

Side effects: Too much fluoride will mottle the teeth and will not give any more strength, so do not exceed the recommended dosage. At recommended dosage there are no known side effects; fluoride is a natural mineral present in many natural water supplies.

DIARRHEA

For occasional loose stools, no medication is required. A clear liquid diet is the first thing to do for any diarrhea. When diarrhea is severe, Kaopectate is the medicine to try at home. When it does not control the diarrhea, stronger agents containing substances such as paregoric may be needed. Protracted diarrhea may require the help of the physician.

Kaopectate

Kaopectate is a combination of a clay-like substance (Kaolin) and pectin, a substance found in apples. The different ingredients have a gelling effect which helps to form a solid stool.

Dosage: For adults, four to eight tablespoons after each bowel movement; for children 3–12, one to four tablespoons; for children below three, call the doctor. With this dosage schedule, more severe diarrhea is treated more vigorously, and minor problems require little medicine.

Side effects: None have been reported.

Paregoric-Containing Preparations: Parapectolin, Parelixir

In addition to a gelling substance, these compounds contain a narcotic (paregoric) which acts to decrease the activity of the digestive tract and thus to slow down the diarrhea. These drugs should be used only when a clear liquid diet and Kaopectate have failed to control very frequent diarrhea, with one or more watery stools per hour.

In most states, these compounds are available without prescriptions, although you must sign for them at the time of purchase.

Dosage: The amount in the table below is given after each loose bowel movement. No more than four doses should be given in any eight-hour period without the approval of your physician.

Age	Dose
1–3 years	½–1½ teaspoons
3–6 years	1½–2 teaspoons
6–12 years	2–3 teaspoons
over 12 years	1–2 tablespoons

Side effects: Narcotic overdosage with paregoric is extremely rare. Drowsiness or nausea occur occasionally, and are indications that the drug should be withdrawn. "Overshoot" can occur, where the diarrhea is controlled so completely that you don't have a bowel movement for a week, so be careful.

Psyllium Hydrophilic Mucilloid: Metamucil, Effersylium

This substance can help both diarrhea and constipation. It draws water into the stool, forms a gel or thick solution, and thus provides bulk. It is a product refined from the psyllium seed. It is not absorbed by the digestive tract but only passes through; thus, it is a natural product, and one with essentially no contraindications and no side effects. With all this going for it, we must admit that it doesn't always work and that a similar effect can probably be obtained by eating enough celery. It has been recommended as a weight reduction aid when taken before meals because it induces a feeling of fullness which may reduce appetite, however, it doesn't seem very effective in this role.

Dosage: One teaspoonful, stirred in a glass of water, taken twice daily is a typical dose. A second glass of water or juice should also be taken. Psyllium is also available in more expensive, individual-dose packets, for times when you don't have a teaspoon. The effervescent versions mix a bit more rapidly and taste better to some.

Side effects: If taken with insufficient water, the gel which is formed may lodge in the esophagus (the tube which leads from mouth to stomach). Sufficient liquid will prevent this problem.

EYE IRRITATIONS

The tear mechanism normally soothes, cleans, and lubricates the eye. Occasionally, the environment can overwhelm this mechanism, or the tear flow may be insufficient. In these cases the eye becomes "tired," feels dry or gritty, and may itch. A number of compounds may be purchased which may aid this problem.

Murine, Visine

There are two general types of eye preparations. One class contains compounds intended to soothe the eye (Murine). Added to the compounds may be substances to shrink blood vessels and thus "get the red out" (Visine). These substances are our old friends the decongestants. Their capacity to soothe is debatable. The use of decongestants to get rid of a bloodshot appearance is totally cosmetic. It is possible that such preparations can actually interfere with the normal healing process, although such occurrence must be unusual.

Methylcellulose Eyedrops

The second group of preparations makes no claims of special soothing effects and contains no decongestants. They are solutions with concentrations like those of the body so that no irritation occurs. Their purpose is to lubricate the eye, to be "artificial tears." These are the preparations preferred by ophthalmologists for minor eye irritation. Methylcellulose eyedrops are an example of this type.

Prefrin

Prefrin lies somewhere between the two; it contains both substances which effectively soothe and lubricate the eye and a decongestant.

Dosage: Use as much and as frequently as needed. You can't use too much, although usually a few drops give just as much relief as a bottleful. If your problem of dry eyes is constant, you should check it out with the doctor, since a major underlying problem could be present. Usually, the symptom of dry eyes lasts only a few hours and is readily relieved. Too much sun, too much wind, or too much dust usually has caused the minor irritation.

Side effects: No serious side effects have been reported. Visine and other drugs containing decongestants tend to sting a bit.

None of these drugs treat infections or injuries or foreign bodies of the eye. In Section II of this book, we give instructions for more severe eye complaints. Refer to: Problem 54, Foreign Body in Eye; Problem 55, Eye Pain; Problem 56, Decreased Vision; Problem 57, Eye Burning, Itching, and Discharge.

HEMORRHOIDS

Zinc Oxide Powders and Creams

These agents aren't magic, but they are good for ordinary problems. The creams soothe the irritated area while the body heals the inflamed vein. They also help toughen the skin over the hemorrhoids so that they are less easily irritated. Don't trap bacteria beneath the creams; apply them after a bath where the area has been carefully cleaned and dried.

Reading the labels: We do not advocate the use of creams with a "-caine" in the list of ingredients because repeated use of these local anesthetics can cause further irritation.

Dosage: Apply as needed, following label directions.

Side effects: Essentially none.

PAIN AND FEVER

Aspirin

Aspirin is the Superdrug. It controls fevers, helps pain, and reduces inflammation. It is the only significant active ingredient in many "over-the-counter" cold and pain remedies, and is the unnamed "ingredient doctors recommend most." Although great quantities of it have been consumed, it nevertheless has an enviable safety record. You can kill yourself with an overdose of aspirin, but it is extremely difficult for an adult.

Aspirin is a bit of an anachronism at the drug counter. If it were developed as a new drug today, it would be available only by prescription. It may be purchased over-the-counter because it was in wide use before the present regulations were in force. Paradoxically, this familiarity with aspirin makes it difficult for the physician. Often, a patient does not accept a suggestion for aspirin, because aspirin is equated with disinterest or neglect on the part of the physician. Or the patient may reject it because of a sensationalistic article describing horrible side effects and implying that aspirin is the cause of much human illness.

The truth in medicine is seldom sensational and is usually consistent with common sense. All drugs are hazardous; aspirin can cause serious problems on occasion, but these are rare if the drug is used appropriately. Usually, a drug alternative to aspirin is more dangerous, has not been studied as completely, and is much more expensive. In addition, the alternative is often not as effective. Prescription pain relievers such as Darvon or codeine (½ grain) are approximately as strong as aspirin.

The claims for excessive purity of expensive preparations of aspirin aren't of much medical relevance. For ourselves, we buy a big jar of the cheapest U.S.P. aspirin at the cut-rate drugstore. If the bottle contains a vinegary odor when opened, the aspirin has begun to deteriorate and should be discarded. Aspirin usually has a shelf life of about three years, although shorter periods are sometimes quoted. (Note: U.S.P. stands for "United States Pharmacopeia." While not an absolute guarantee that the drug is the best, it does mean that the drug has met certain standards in composition and physical characteristics. The same is true of the designation N.F., which stands for "National Formulary.")

Dosage: In adults, the standard dose for pain relief is two tablets taken every three to four hours as required. The maximum effect occurs in about two hours. Each standard tablet is five grains, or 300 milligrams, or 0.3 grams. If you use a nonstandard concoction, you will have to do the arithmetic to calculate equivalent doses. The terms "extra-strength," "arthritis pain formula," and the like indicate a greater amount of aspirin per tablet. This is medically trivial. You can take more tablets of the cheaper aspirin and still save money. When you read that a product "contains more of the ingredient that doctors recommend most" you may be sure that the product contains a little bit more aspirin per tablet; perhaps 325 to 350 mgm instead of 300.

Here are some hints for good aspirin usage. Aspirin treats symptoms; it does not cure problems. Thus, for symptoms such as headache or muscle pain or menstrual cramps, don't take it unless you hurt. On the other hand, for control of fever you will be more comfortable if you repeat the dose every three to four hours during the day, since this prevents the fever from bouncing up and down like a yo-yo. For fever, the afternoon and evening are the worst, so try not to miss a dose during these hours. If you need aspirin for relief from some symptom over a prolonged period, check the symptom with your doctor. Pain relief is little different if you increase the dose, and you are more likely to irritate your stomach, so stick with the standard dose even if you still have some discomfort. The same holds for fever. For other ways of lowering fever, see page 59.

For control of inflammation, as in serious arthritis, the dose of aspirin must be high, often 16 to 20 tablets daily, and must be continued over a prolonged period. A physician should monitor such treatment; it is relatively safe but problems sometimes occur.

In children, a dose of about one grain (60 mgm) for each year of age is appropriate, and leads to an adult dose for children over 10 years. Children's aspirin comes in 1.25 grain (75 mgm) tablets which taste good; please do not allow them to be taken for candy by a small child.

Aspirin can be given as a rectal suppository if vomiting prevents taking medication by mouth. The doses are the same as if given by mouth. Five and ten grain suppositories may be cut to allow smaller doses for smaller people. Suppositories will irritate the rectum if used repeatedly, so try to limit their use to two or three doses. These suppositories require a prescription.

Side effects: Frequently aspirin will upset the stomach or cause ringing in the ears. If the stomach is upset, try taking the aspirin a half-hour after meals, when the food in the stomach will act as a buffer. Coated aspirin (such as Ecotrin or A.S.A. Enseals) will almost totally protect the stomach. However, some people do not digest the coated aspirin, and so receive no benefit. Buffering is sometimes added to aspirin to protect the stomach, and may help a little. If you take a lot of aspirin and desire a buffered preparation, we recommend a nonabsorbable antacid (as in Ascriptin) to be used in combination rather than an absorbable antacid, as in most buffered aspirins. Nonabsorbable antacids are much easier on your system. Over the short-term it makes little difference, and there is controversy as to whether any of the buffering works anyway. If the ears ring, reduce the dose; you are taking too much and will do just as well with a bit less.

Rarely, asthma, nasal polyps, deafness, serious bleeding from the digestive tract, ulcers, and other major problems have been associated with aspirin. Such problems are unusual and almost always disappear after the aspirin is stopped. Conversely, some studies suggest that aspirin might be good treatment for hardening of the arteries; but this has by no means been proven.

Aspirin comes in combination with many other remedies not described in this book, most frequently caffeine and phenacetin ("APC Tabs"). Some scientists think these agents increase the pain-killing effects; others dispute this. They do increase the side effects, and we find little use for them. Do not use products with caffeine if you have heart trouble or difficulty sleeping; do not use products with phenacetin over a long period because kidney damage has been reported.

Acetaminophen: Tylenol, Datril, Liquiprin, Tempra

Aspirin is the drug of first choice for treatment of minor pains and minor fever. Acetaminophen, available in several brand-name preparations, is next. It is slightly less predictable than aspirin, somewhat less powerful, and does not have the antiinflammatory action which makes aspirin so valuable in treatment of arthritis and other diseases. On the other hand, it does not cause ringing in the ears or upset the stomach—common side effects with aspirin. Many pediatricians feel that acetaminophen is preferable in children for these reasons. In the British Commonwealth, this drug is known as paracetamol.

Dosage: Acetaminophen is used in doses identical to those of aspirin. For adults, two five-grain tablets every three to four hours are standard. In children, one grain per year of age every four hours is satisfactory. There is no reason ever to exceed these doses, since there is no additional benefit by higher amounts. Acetaminophen is available in liquid preparations which are palatable for small children. These are usually administered by a dropper, and the package insert gives the amount for each age of child.

Side effects: These are seldom seen. If you suspect a side effect, call your physician. A variety of very rare toxic effects have been reported, but none are definitely related to the use of this drug. Like aspirin, acetaminophen comes in multiple combination products which offer little advantage.

PAIN AND FEVER: CHILDHOOD

The principles and drugs used to control minor pain and fever in the child are the same as in the adult, but there are important differences in the importance of treatment and in the method of administration. In the child, fever comes on more rapidly and may rise much higher, even with a minor virus. The fever must be controlled; high fever can lead to a frightening temporary epilepsy, with seizures or "fits." Thus, while control of the fever in an adult is principally for the comfort of the patient, fever control in the child actually prevents serious complications. It can be difficult to get the small sick child to take medication, thus different methods of administration are sometimes needed.

If the child has a rash, a stiff neck, trouble breathing, is lethargic, or looks very ill, call or visit the doctor. Be particularly careful with children under one year of age. Phone advice is graciously available in most areas; don't hesitate to call if you have a question. Many times the child, despite a high fever, will look fine and not even be very irritable. In such cases, treatment and observation at home are adequate. Physicians frequently prefer a phone call to a visit, because, if the visit can be avoided, other children in the waiting room or office are not exposed to the virus.

Liquid Acetaminophen or Aspirin

Many pediatricians prefer acetaminophen or sodium salicylate over aspirin for the small child, principally because these agents have less chance of causing stomach upset. The liquid preparations are easier to administer and are better tolerated by the stomach. (If vomiting makes it impossible to keep even these liquid medicines down, the use of rectal suppositories of aspirin can be very helpful.)

Dosage: For liquid aspirin or acetaminophen preparations, follow the label advice. Administer every four hours. During the period from noon to midnight, awaken the child if necessary. After midnight, the fever will usually break by itself and become less of a problem, so if you miss a dose it is less important. But check the temperature at least once during the night to make sure. Remember, these drugs only last about four hours in the body, and you must keep repeating the dose or you will lose the effect. Some pediatricians recommend alternating aspirin and acetaminophen at two-hour intervals for high fevers.

Aspirin Rectal Suppositories

Rectal aspirin suppositories, unfortunately, are available only by prescription in most localities. The dose is the same as by mouth; one grain (60 milligrams) per year of age per four hours. This formula works up to age 10, then use adult doses. One-grain suppositories are manufactured but are sometimes difficult to find at a store. If necessary, cut the larger five grain suppositories down to make an approximate equivalent to the dose needed. Use a warm knife and cut them lengthwise. Ask your physician for a prescription for rectal aspirin suppositories on a routine visit if you can't get them over-the-counter. Keep them in stock at home. Use them only when vomiting prevents retention of any oral intake, and do not exceed three doses for any one illness without contacting your physician.

Use of suppositories confuses many parents. The idea is to allow the medicine to be absorbed through the mucus membranes of the rectum. Remove the wrapper before use. When inserting the suppository, firm but gentle pressure will cause the muscles to relax around the rectum. Be patient. In small children, the buttocks may need to be held or taped together to prevent expulsion of the suppository.

Side effects: Rectal aspirin can irritate the rectum and cause local bleeding; therefore it should only be used if the ordinary routes of administration are impossible—even then, if more than two or three doses seem to be required, call your physician for advice.

Other Measures

Cool or lukewarm baths are also useful in keeping a fever down. During the bath, wet the hair as well. Keep the patient in a cool room, wearing little or no clothing.

POISONING

To Induce Vomiting: Syrup of Ipecac

Keep this traditional remedy handy if you have small children. With most poisonings, promptly inducing vomiting will empty the stomach of any poison which has not already been absorbed. Do not use any agent to cause vomiting if the poison swallowed is a petroleum-based compound or is a strong acid or a strong alkali (see Section II, Problem 12, Poisoning).

It is far better to keep toxic chemicals out of a child's reach than to have to use ipecac. When you buy ipecac, use the purchase as a reminder to check the house for toxic chemicals which a child might reach, and remove them to a safer place. However, if your child does swallow something, the sooner the stomach is emptied the milder will be the problem, with the exceptions listed above. There is no time to buy ipecac after your child has swallowed poison; you should have it on hand—just in case it's ever needed.

Dosage: A tablespoonful may suffice for a small child, two are necessary for older children and adults. Follow with as much warm water as can be given, until vomiting occurs. Repeat the dose in fifteen minutes if you haven't had any results.

Side effects: This is an uncomfortable medication, but not hazardous unless vomiting causes vomited material to be thrown down the windpipe into the lungs. This will cause a severe pneumonia; so do not induce vomiting in a patient who is unconscious or nearly unconscious, and do not cause vomiting of flammable materials which can be inhaled into the lung and cause damage. A call to the local poison control center should be made in any potentially severe poisoning. In this setting, giving ipecac on the way to the hospital may be helpful and even can be lifesaving. But the experts at the poison control center can tell you for sure.

SKIN DRYNESS

Moisturizing Creams and Lotions: Lubriderm, Vaseline, Corn Huskers, Nivea

When it comes to the various kinds of artificial materials which human beings apply to their skin in the attempt to temporarily improve its appearance or to retard its aging there is little to be said. The various claims are not scientifically based, and long-term benefits have not been demonstrated. In some areas, harm has been postulated instead of benefit.

Sometimes, dry skin can actually cause symptoms and becomes a medical problem. Then, something is needed which is safe, nontoxic, nonallergenic, and which provides relief. Of products available over-the-counter, Lubriderm, Vaseline, or Corn Huskers lotion are as good as any. Nivea is effective but an occasional person is sensitive to the lanolin it contains. Remember that you may be contributing to the drying by bathing or exposure to detergents. Decreasing the frequency of baths or showers, wearing gloves when working with cleansing agents, and other similar measures are more important than using any lotion or cream.

Dosage: Per product label.

Side effects: Essentially none except for the rare lanolin sensitivity mentioned above.

SKIN FUNGUS

Antifungal Preparations: Tinactin, Selsun, Desenex

Fungal infections of the skin are not serious and treatment is not urgent. In general, the fungus needs moist undisturbed areas to grow and will often disappear with regular cleansing, drying, and application of a powder to keep the area dry. Cleansing should be performed twice daily.

If you need a medication, there are effective nontoxic agents available. For athlete's foot we like first one of the zinc undecylenate creams or powders, such as Desenex. In difficult cases, tolnaftate (Tinactin) is very effective. This agent is useful for almost all skin fungus problems, but is more expensive. For superficial fungus infection, particularly those causing patchy loss of skin color, selenium sulfide (Selsun Blue) is often quickly effective.

Dosage: For athlete's foot, use as directed on the label. For other skin problems selenium sulfide is available by prescription in a 2½% strength. Over-the-counter, a 1% solution is available as Selsun Blue shampoo. Use the shampoo as a cream and let it dry on the lesions; repeat several times a day to make up for the weaker strength.

Side effects: There are very few. Selenium sulfide can burn the skin if used to excess, so decrease application if you notice any irritation. Selenium may discolor hair and will stain clothes. Be very careful around the eyes with any of these products. And *don't* take them by mouth.

Sunscreen Products: Pre-Sun, Block-Out, Paba-Film, Pabonal

Dermatologists continually remind us that sun is bad for the skin. Exposure to the sun accelerates the aging process and increases chances of skin cancer. Advertisements, on the other hand, continually extol the virtues of a suntan, and as a nation we spend much of our youth trying to achieve a pleasing skin tone, with disregard for the later consequences of solar radiation. The sunscreen agents can be used to prevent burning but to allow tanning. Where the skin is unusually sensitive to the sun's effects, a more complete block of the rays is best. Partial blocking of the sun's rays is afforded by Block-Out and Paba-Film, while Pabonal and Pre-Sun block out virtually all rays. Suntan lotions which are not sunscreen agents block relatively little solar radiation.

Dosage: Apply evenly to exposed areas of skin as directed on the label.

Side effects: Very rare skin irritation or allergy.

SPRAINS

Elastic Bandages

Elastic (Ace) bandages find periodic use in any family. Probably you will need both a narrow and a broader width. If problems are recurrent, the circular bandages designed specifically for knee and ankle are sometimes more convenient. All of these bandages primarily provide gentle support, but also act to reduce swelling. Elastic bandages should be used if they make the injured part feel better. The support given is minimal and re-injury is possible despite the bandage. Thus it is not a substitute for a splint, a cast, or a proper adhesive-tape dressing when these are needed. Perhaps the most important function of these bandages is as a reminder to you that you have a problem so that you are less likely to reinjure the part.

Dosage: Support should be continued well past the time of active discomfort to allow complete healing and to help prevent reinjury; this usually requires about six weeks. During the latter part of this period the bandages may be used only for activities where stress on the injured part is likely. Remember, reinjury is still possible with these bandages.

Side effects: The simple elastic bandage can cause trouble when not properly applied. Problems arise because the bandage is applied too tightly, and circulation in the limb beyond the bandage is impaired. The bandage should be firm and not tight. The limb should not swell, hurt, or be cooler beyond the bandage. There should not be any blueness or purple color to the limb. When wrapping the bandage, start at the most distant area to be bandaged and work toward the body, making each loop a little looser than the one before. Thus, a knee bandage should be tighter below the knee than above, and an ankle bandage tighter on the foot than on the lower leg. Many people think that because a bandage is elastic it must be stretched. This is not the case. The stretching is for when you move. Simply wrap the bandage as you would a roll of gauze.

UPSET STOMACH

Absorbable Antacids: Baking Soda, Alka-Seltzer Gold, Tums

The main ingredient in these products is sodium bicarbonate, and this will neutralize acid, at least in a test tube. In the human stomach, its action is not so clear. For one thing, it may be absorbed through the walls of the stomach, thus not helping with the acid problem there and, in large doses, upsetting the body's own chemistry. More important, there may be "rebound" after taking sodium bicarbonate; that is, the stomach may be stimulated to secrete more acid. This, of course, only adds to the problem and may be one reason that any relief is short. For these reasons, we prefer the nonabsorbable antacids.

Nonabsorbable Antacids: Maalox, Gelusil, Mylanta, Alugel, Wingel, Riopan

The nonabsorbable antacids are an important part of the home pharmacy. They help neutralize stomach acid and thus decrease heartburn, ulcer pain, gas pains, and stomach upset. Since they are not absorbed by the body, they do not usually upset the acid-base balance of the body and are quite safe.

Almost all of these antacids are available in both liquid and tablet form. For most purposes, the liquid form is superior. It coats more of the surface area of the gullet and stomach than the tablets do. Indeed, if not well chewed, the tablets may be almost worthless. Still, the pressure of work or play can make a bottle a cumbersome companion, and a few tablets in the shirt pocket or purse may help out with midday doses.

Reading the labels: Nonabsorbable antacids contain magnesium or aluminum, or both. As a general rule, magnesium causes diarrhea and aluminum causes constipation. Different brands are slightly different mixtures of salts of these two metals, designed to avoid both diarrhea and constipation. A few brands also contain calcium, which is mildly constipating; in general the calcium-containing preparations should be avoided.

Different products differ in taste. While there are some differences in potency, most people will ultimately select that particular antacid which doesn't upset their bowels in either direction and has a taste they can tolerate. Keep trying different brands until you are happy.

Dosage: Two tablespoons (30cc) or two tablets, well-chewed, is the standard adult dose. One-half as much for 6 to 12 year olds, and a quarter as much for children three to six. The frequency of the dose depends upon the severity of the problem. For stomach upset or heartburn, one or two doses may often suffice. For gastritis, several days of several doses each may be needed. For ulcers, six weeks or more may be needed, with the medication taken as frequently as every hour or so; this type of program should be supervised by a physician.

Side effects: In general, only the effect on the bowel movements is a problem. Maalox tends to loosen the stools a bit, Mylanta and Gelusil to be about average, and Alugel and Aludrox (with more aluminum) to be more constipating. Adjust the brand as needed. Check with your doctor before using these compounds if you have kidney disease, heart disease, or high blood pressure. Some brands contain significant quantities of salt and should be avoided by persons on a low-salt diet. Riopan has the lowest salt content of the popular brands.

WARTS

Wart Removers: Compound W, Vergo

Warts are a funny little problem. The capricious way in which they form and disappear has led to countless myths and home therapies. They can be surgically removed, burned off, or frozen off, but they also will go away by themselves or after treatment by hypnosis. Warts are caused by a virus and are a reaction to a minor local viral infection. If you get one, you are likely to get more. When one disappears, the others often follow.

Chemicals available over-the-counter for treatment of warts are moderately effective. They contain a mild skin irritant. By repeated application, the top layers of the wart are slowly burned off, and eventually the virus is destroyed.

Dosage: Apply repeatedly, as directed on the product label. Persistence is necessary.

Side effects: These products are effective by being caustic to the skin, therefore be careful you apply them only to the wart, and be very careful around eyes or mouth.

WOUNDS (Minor)

Adhesive Tape/Bandages

Bandages really don't "make it better," and sometimes leaving a minor wound open to the air is preferable to covering it. Still, it wouldn't be a home medical shelf without a tin of assorted adhesive bandages. They are useful for covering tender blisters, keeping dirt out of wounds, and keeping the edges of a cut together. To the patient, they frequently find value keeping the wound out of sight and thus are of cosmetic importance. You need also adhesive tape and gauze, in order to fashion larger bandages.

Dosage: For small cuts and sores, use a bandage from the tin. Usually a day or so is long enough; change the bandage if you wish to use it longer. For cuts, apply the bandage perpendicular to the cut, and draw the skin toward the cut from both sides to relax skin tension before applying the bandage. The bandage should then act to keep the edges together during healing. For larger injuries, make a bandage from a roll of sterile gauze or from sterile 2 x 2" or 4 x 4" gauze pads, and tape it in place, firmly, with adhesive tape. Change daily. If you see white fat protruding from the cut, see the doctor.

Side effects: If the wound isn't clean when you cover it with a bandage, you may hide a developing infection from early discovery. Get it clean and keep it clean. The bandage should be changed if it becomes wet. Many people are allergic to adhesive tape; they should use one of the paper tapes which are nonallergenic. If adhesive tape is left on for a week or so it will irritate almost anyone's skin, so give the skin a rest. Some patients leave a bandage on too long because they are afraid of the pain as they remove the bandage— particularly if there is hair caught in the tape! For painless removal, soak the adhesive tape in nail polish remover (applied from the back) for five minutes. This will dissolve the adhesive and release both skin and hair.

Antiseptics: Hydrogen Peroxide/Iodine

A dirty wound often becomes infected; if dirt or foreign bodies are trapped beneath the skin they can fester and delay wound healing. At the time of a wound only a few germs are introduced, but they may multiply over several days to a very large number. The purposes of an antiseptic are to remove the dirt and to kill the germs. Most of the time, the cleansing action is the more important because many antiseptic solutions such as hydrogen peroxide, merthiolate, Zephiran, or mercurochrome really aren't very good at killing germs. We think that hydrogen peroxide, which foams and cleans as you work it in the wound, is a good cleansing agent and that iodine is a good agent with which to kill germs. Scrupulous attention to the cleaning of a wound initially and the scrubbing out of any imbedded dirt particles are crucial to good healing. Do this even though it hurts and bleeds. For small clean cuts we use soap and water followed by iodine and then by soap and water again. For larger wounds we like hydrogen peroxide with vigorous scrubbing. Betadine is a nonstinging iodine preparation. First-aid sprays are a waste of money.

Dosage: Hydrogen peroxide should not be used in strengths greater than 3%, so watch out for bottles sold at higher strength for bleaching hair. Most hydrogen peroxide is sold at the 3% strength and may be used full strength. Pour it on and scrub with a rough cloth. Wash off and repeat. Keep on until there is no dirt visible beneath the level of the skin. If you can't get it clean, go to the doctor.

Iodine is painted or wiped onto the wound and the surrounding area. Wash it off within a few minutes, leaving a trace of the iodine color on the skin.

Side effects: Iodine will burn the skin if left on full strength, so be careful. Hydrogen peroxide is safe to the skin, but can bleach hair and clothing, so try not to spill it. Some people are allergic to iodine; discontinue use if you get a rash.

Soaking Agent: Sodium Bicarbonate (Baking Soda)

Sodium bicarbonate (baking soda, $NaHCO_3$) is a very useful household chemical. It has three principal medical uses. As a strong solution, it will draw fluid and swelling out of a wound, and will act to soak and clean the wound at the same time. As a weaker solution, it acts to soothe the skin and to reduce itching; thus it is helpful in conditions ranging from sunburn to poison oak to chicken pox. If taken by mouth it serves as an antacid and may help heartburn or stomach upset.

Dosage: (1) For soaking a wound: one tablespoon to a cup of warm water. If a finger or toe is injured, it may be placed in the cup; for other wounds a wash cloth should be saturated with the solution and placed over the wound as a compress. Generally, a wound should be soaked for 5 to 10 minutes at a time, three times a day. If the skin is puckered and "water-logged" after the soak, it has been soaked too long. A cellophane or plastic wrap may be placed over the cloth compress to retain heat and moisture longer. (2) For soothing the skin: from two tablespoons to a half-cup in a bath of warm water, blotted gently after the bath and allowed to dry on the skin; repeated as often as necessary. (3) As an antacid: one teaspoonful in a glass of water, every four hours as needed—but only very occasionally (see Antacids).

Side effects: There are none as long as the baking soda is only applied to the skin. If you take it by mouth, watch out for two things. First, there is a lot of sodium in it, and if you have heart trouble or high blood pressure or are on a low-salt diet you can get into a lot of trouble. Secondly, if you take it for many months on a regular basis, there is some evidence that it may result in calcium deposits in the kidneys and in kidney damage. As an antacid it is "absorbable," and is thus more dangerous than antacids which are not absorbed by the intestine.

VITAMIN DEFICIENCY

Vitamin Preparations

Americans are said to have the most expensive urine in the world. Much of its added worth comes from unneeded vitamins which are excreted unchanged in the urine and cannot aid the body. Vitamins are chemically known as coenzymes. They are essential to normal function but are required in only very small amounts. With an ordinary diet, many times the required amounts of vitamins are provided. Only in the severe alcoholic or in the person with an unusually limited diet is vitamin supplementation required.

Megavitamin doses, providing many times the known requirements for vitamin C, vitamin E, and other vitamins have been advocated by a few. Considering the biological role of vitamins in enzyme systems, the available vitamin supply to primitive societies, and the forces of evolution, it is difficult to conceive of a role for such extra vitamin therapy. Extra vitamins have never been shown to decrease colds, improve the sex life, or restore lost energy. Continuing investigations into the role of vitamins is underway at many institutions. Pending final results, it is important for you to know that doctors, who can get vitamins free, almost never take them. Your authors do not take vitamins, nor do they give vitamins to their families.

Unless a physician documents a vitamin deficiency and recommends a supplement, use of vitamins is entirely optional. It's your money. If you must buy, select the cheaper "house" brands which do not advertise heavily.

Dosage: As specified by a physician for the individual's use.

Side effects: Vitamin A and vitamin D can cause severe problems when excessively large doses are taken. Vitamin C is theoretically toxic when taken in large doses but has not yet proved much of a practical problem. Other vitamins have not been as well studied, but no serious side effects are known.

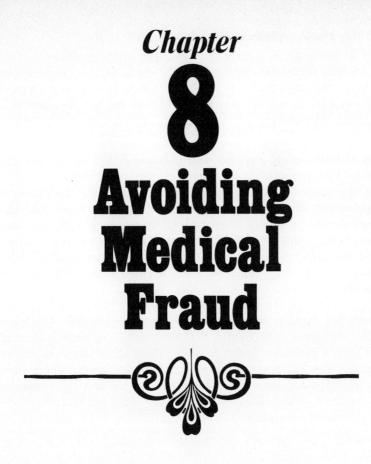

Chapter
8
Avoiding Medical Fraud

At least two billion dollars yearly are spent on frauds, hoaxes, and false cures. You probably contribute to this windfall. When you buy over-the-counter drugs as a result of TV advertisements, take massive amounts of the vitamin-of-the-month, or send away for "cures" advertised in the back of magazines, you are paying part of this bill. You are being hustled.

You can recognize a hustle. There are four easy questions, one or more of which will usually identify the dishonest marketer. The questions are: What is the motive of the marketer? What are the claims made? Do experts use the service? Does the service make sense? Let's look at these questions.

What is the motive of the marketer?

Make some rough estimates of the proposed service as a business. Does it look like a revolving-door operation, where people walk in one door with their money and soon thereafter leave without it? What is the average fee paid by the customer? How many patients are seen each hour? The product of these two numbers represents the hourly income of the operation. If this gross amount exceeds one hundred dollars per professional employee, watch out.

What Are the Promises and Claims Made?

Vague? Misleading? A typical advertisement urges purchase of a product "containing an ingredient recommended by doctors." This is clearly intended to deceive; the advertiser knows that if the ingredient were named, you would recognize it to be relatively ineffective for the problem or readily available at less expense.

Beware of testimonials, coupons, and guarantees: If a product or service is advertised by testimonial, it is probably of marginal value or lower. A testimonial may consist of "before and after" pictures. It may be a story related by a presumed patient relating success with the treatment. On occasion, testimonials will be totally fabricated. However, even if the testimonial is accurate, it provides no reliable information. You are not interested in whether the proposed service has *ever* helped *anyone,* you are interested in whether it is *likely to help you.* There is an important difference in these statements.

Coupons are another clue to bad services. Worthwhile treatments are not marketed through magazine and newspaper coupons. Guarantees in medicine are almost a guarantee that the product or service is worthless. In medicine, a guarantee is not possible. There are always exceptions; and always, the possibility of unfortunate results. No worthwhile medical service is accompanied by a guarantee. Thus it isn't that the guarantee will not be honored (which is probably also the case) but that the offer itself strongly suggests a suspicious product.

Do experts in the field use the service?

Does your doctor take the vitamin you are considering? Does his family? Do arthritis doctors with arthritis wear copper bracelets? Do cancer doctors use laetrile when their mother or wife has cancer? Doctors (and their families) get cancer and other diseases just as frequently as anybody else. If any treatment had the remotest chance of benefiting one of these serious conditions, the physician would utilize that product or service. In point of fact, physicians do *not* use these marginal services. Doctors have decreased their cigarette smoking. They have taken up jogging and other regular forms of exercise. They have not endorsed megavitamin therapy, diet fads, and other popular fancies by their own use.

Who, if anyone, endorses the service? Is it endorsed by a national professional organization? Is it endorsed by a national consumer organization? Direct product endorsement by such organizations is rare, but of great value if present. Endorsement of toothpaste containing stannous fluoride by the American Dental Association is an example. Consumers Union may be relied upon for thoughtful discussions of the medical issues of the day.

Does the proposed service make sense?

This is the final test. Frequently, frauds and false cures occur because no one really asks whether common sense approves. Do you really think that creams will significantly improve your bust line? Or that you can lose weight only in the hips? Or that a vitamin will help your sex life? Or that a lamb's embryo will keep you young? By definition, a false cure has a false rationale advanced. This rationale is often weak and easily identified as such.

Three Examples

Three of the oldest and largest medical rackets victimize people with the problems of obesity, arthritis, or cancer.

Overweight people appear particularly willing victims for the fringe health entrepreneur. As we noted in Chapter 1, successful weight control is achieved gradually, through moderate programs, and must be sustained for a lifetime. A weight-loss program has merit when it projects its program for a prolonged period. There is negligible medical benefit (and quite possibly harm) in weight loss which occurs abruptly and lasts only a few weeks or months. Individuals with a significant weight problem face a very difficult task requiring intense commitment, long-term discipline, and considerable emotional distress. We applaud the courage of those who undertake such a program and the fortitude of those able to maintain an important but difficult task.

The fraudulent approach is to promise a short-cut. A gadget of some type, massage, a miracle diet, an appetite suppressant, a food supplement, or some other mechanism is promoted as a way to "lose weight fast and easy." "Fast" and "easy" do not describe safe and effective weight loss programs.

The facts are relatively straightforward. Most overweight people do not succeed in losing weight and maintaining a steady desirable level under *any* program. The best results have been obtained under medically supervised programs, and with reputable long-term programs such as "Weight Watchers." Spot-reducing (reduction of fat at one particular point in the body such as the hips or legs) does *not* work. Massage is not an effective way to lose weight. Appetite suppressants have not been successful over the long term. There is frequently a brief period of weight loss with any technique promoted. An occasional success may be seen with almost any program, but *it is the individual and not the fad* that is responsible for the improvement.

Arthritis is another ideal subject for exploitation. These conditions are chronic and often discouraging. A widespread impression exists that arthritis cannot be treated by traditional medicine. The tragedy of false fads in arthritis is aggravated, however, because *good treatment is available* for almost all patients. Patients unnecessarily crippled by having avoided sound, established medical approaches are regularly seen. In the area of arthritis, the fourth test for recognizing a hustle is most frequently of use: Does it make sense? Diet for arthritis? You can understand a diet for losing weight, but what has that got to do with pain in the joints? Vinegar and honey for arthritis? More than a little strange. Copper bracelets? Really.

A legend persists that other countries have better drugs for arthritis than the United States. It is true that the Food and Drug Administration has rather carefully limited approval of new therapies for arthritis. There have been, at most points in recent years, several drugs available in Mexico, Canada, and Europe which are not yet licensed in the United States. However, none of these drugs is a major addition to existing therapy. The position of the Food and Drug Administration has been to insure as carefully as possible the safety of new medications before allowing them to enter the market. There are no magical new drugs.

The legend of dramatic new treatments, however, has led to fraudulent medical operations just over the Mexican border. (Such operations should not be confused with the very fine medicine available at many locations in Mexico.) These "arthritis mills" attract patients from the United States, who come long distances to be seen briefly and return to the United States with bags and boxes full of medications. Patients are told a variety of things about these medications; but usually, it is suggested that they are being given drugs not available in the United States. We have had occasion to analyze the contents of such medications, and the active ingredient has uniformly been a drug related to cortisone. In addition, a drug called phenylbutazone is often present in combination. These drugs are hazardous and have resulted in fatalities in patients treated in these "arthritis mills." Ill-conceived therapies with such drugs often make patients feel better over the first few days and weeks; such short-term improvement is what keeps the waiting rooms full. Over the longer term, increased disability and possibly death will result. Common sense suggests that the best medical care in the world is unlikely to be found in Mexican border towns. When you suspend common sense, you can lose more than money.

Acupuncture has received great publicity and is under intensive evaluation as a treatment for arthritis. The early studies suggest a minor effect in pain relief, rather less strong than aspirin. However, final information is not yet available. Other fad cures are already definitely discredited. Corticosteroids and cortisone are seldom required in arthritis and, if used for a prolonged period, are almost always detrimental.

Cancer is the area of the cruelest hoaxes. In some cases, where cancer has already spread throughout the body, orthodox medicine cannot help the patient very much. In this setting, the vultures move in. "What have you got to lose?" is their call. The answer is that you may lose *courage*, *dignity*, and *money*. The problem however is that you have nothing to gain.

Cancer is not one but many diseases, requiring many different approaches to treatment. Very effective treatment is available for some cancers, and new techniques are being applied as fast as they can be proven. The great majority of cancer patients can be helped by present medical treatment. The proportion of cures has passed one-quarter and is moving toward one-half. Many agencies and many patients are working very hard to contribute to knowledge in cancer. This is a sophisticated field, with many minds working toward solutions. It is highly unlikely that significant discoveries will come in the form of apricot pits or horse serum. In our own experience we have seen hundreds of patients take dozens of different false "cures"; none have appeared to benefit.

You are hustled because you want to believe. Your wish that the claims might be true does not make them become so. In the theater, you may attempt to cultivate a "willful suspension of disbelief." In medicine, you must constantly strive to *retain* this critical faculty.

Section
II

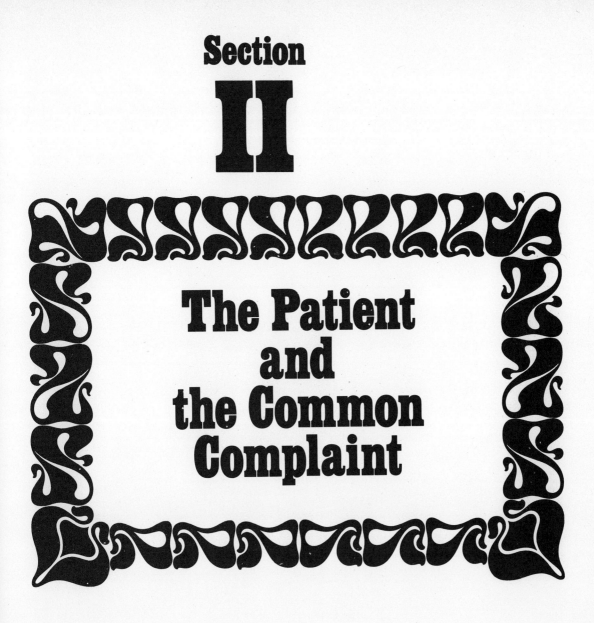

The Patient
and
the Common
Complaint

A
How to Use
This Section

In this section, you will find general information and instruction charts for nearly seventy common medical problems. The *general information* on the lefthand page will give you background on a specific medical problem; also, it will provide instructions for home treatment, as well as what to expect at the doctor's office, if you go. The *charts* on the righthand page will help you decide whether to use home treatment or to consult a physician. To gain the most benefit from this part of the book, use these simple guidelines:

Emergencies. Before dealing with any medical problem at home, the first question to ask is whether or not emergency action is necessary. Often the answer is obvious. The great majority of complaints are quickly recognized as minor. The true emergency is hard to ignore. The information in Emergencies, page 77, presents a common sense approach to several problems which require immediate action. All instruction charts assume that emergency symptoms have been considered first.

Finding the right chart for your medical problem. Determine your "chief complaint" or symptom—for instance, a cough, an earache, or chest pains—and look it up in the Table of Contents, or in the Index, then turn to the appropriate page.

Multiple problems. If you have more than one problem you may have to use more than one instruction chart. For example, if you have a bad sore throat, a slight cough, and a runny nose, look up your most serious complaint first, then the next most serious, etc. You may notice some duplication of questions in the instruction charts, especially when the symptoms are closely related. If you use more than one chart, take the most "conservative" advice; if one chart recommends home treatment and another advises a visit to the physician, then go to the doctor.

Using the charts. First, read all of the general information under your particular problem, then go to the instruction charts. Start at the top and follow the arrows. Skipping around may result in errors. Each question assumes that all questions before have been answered. The general information under the medical problem will help you understand the questions in the chart. If this general material is ignored, a question may be misinterpreted and the wrong course of action selected.

If the chart indicates home treatment. Don't assume that an instruction to use home treatment guarantees that the problem is trivial and may be ignored. Home therapy must be approached conscientiously if it is to work. If over-the-counter medicines are suggested, look them up in the Index and read about dosage and side effects in Chapter 7 before you use them.

There are times when home treatment is not effective despite conscientious application, and, in these cases, a physician should be consulted. The length of time you should wait before consulting a doctor is indicated in the general information for each problem. The home treatment we include in these pages is what most physicians recommend as a first approach to these problems. If it doesn't work, think the problem through again. If you are seriously worried about your condition, call the doctor.

If the chart indicates that you should consult a physician. This does not necessarily mean that the illness is serious or dangerous. Often you are directed to the doctor because a physical examination needs to be performed or because certain facilities of the physician's office are needed. The chart will refer you to a physician with different levels of urgency. "See physician now." means right away. "See physician today." indicates that the visit should be the same day. "Make appointment with physician" means a less urgent situation; the visit should be scheduled, but may take place any time during the next few days. Sometimes, we will give you the medical terminology related to a specific problem. With this information, you will be able to "translate" the terms your doctor may use during your visit or telephone call.

With these guidelines, you will be able to use the instruction charts to quickly locate the information you need, while not burdening yourself with information that you do not require. Look over the charts for several complaints; you will quickly get the knack of finding the answers you need.

B
Emergencies

Emergencies require prompt action, not panic. What action you should take depends on the facilities available and the nature of the problem. If there are massive injuries or if the patient is unconscious, you must get help immediately. Go to the emergency room if it is close. If it isn't, you can often obtain help over the phone by calling an emergency room or the Rescue Squad. This is especially important if you think that someone in your family has swallowed poison.

The most important thing is to *be prepared* to go or to phone. Record the phone numbers of the nearest emergency facility, poison control center, and rescue squad in the front of this book. Know the best way to reach the emergency room by car. Develop these procedures *before* an actual emergency arises.

When to call an ambulance. Usually, the slowest way to reach a medical facility is by ambulance. It must go both ways and often is not twice as fast as a private car. If the patient can readily move or be moved, and a private car is available, use the car and have someone call ahead. The ambulance is expensive and may be needed more urgently at another location, so engage it with care.

The ambulance brings with it a trained crew, who know how to lift a patient to minimize chance of further injury. Oxygen is usually available; splints and bandages are carried; and, in some instances, life-saving resuscitation may be employed en route to the hospital. Thus, the patient who is gravely ill, who has a back or head injury, or who is severely short of breath may benefit from care afforded by the ambulance attendants.

In our experience, ambulances are often used as expensive taxis. The type of accident or illness, the facilities available, and the distance involved are all important factors in deciding whether an ambulance should be used.

The instruction charts in the rest of this book assume that no emergency signs are present. These signs "overrule" the charts and dictate that medical help be sought immediately. Be familiar with the following emergency signs:

Major injury. Common sense tells us that the patient with the obviously broken leg or the large chest wound deserves immediate attention. Emergency facilities exist to take care of major injuries. They should be used, and promptly.

Unconsciousness. The patient who is unconscious needs emergency care immediately.

Active bleeding. Most cuts will stop bleeding if pressure is applied to the wound. Unless the bleeding is obviously minor, a wound which continues to bleed despite the application of pressure requires attention in order to prevent unnecessary loss of blood. The average adult can tolerate the loss of several cups of blood with little ill effect, but children can tolerate only smaller amounts, proportional to their body size. Remember that active and vigorous bleeding can almost always be controlled by the application of pressure directly to the wound and that this is the most important part of first aid for such wounds.

Stupor or drowsiness. A decreased level of mental activity, short of unconsciousness, is termed "stupor." A practical way of telling if the severity of stupor or drowsiness warrants urgent treatment is to note the patient's ability to answer questions. If the patient is not sufficiently awake to answer questions concerning what has happened, then urgent action is necessary. Children are difficult to judge, but the child who cannot be aroused needs immediate attention.

Disorientation. Within medicine, disorientation is described in terms of time, place, and person. This simply means that a patient cannot tell the date, the location, or who he or she is. The person who does not know his or her own identity is in a more difficult state than the person who cannot give the correct date. Disorientation may be part of a variety of illnesses and is especially common when a high fever is present. The patient who previously has been alert and then becomes disoriented and confused deserves immediate medical attention.

Shortness of breath. Shortness of breath is described more extensively in Problem 52. As a general rule, a patient deserves immediate attention if he is short of breath even though resting. However, in young adults the most frequent cause of shortness of breath at rest is the hyperventilation syndrome, Problem 46, which is not a serious concern. Nevertheless, if it cannot be confidently determined that shortness of breath is due to the hyperventilation syndrome, then the only reasonable course of action is to seek immediate aid.

Cold sweats. Sweating is the normal response to elevated temperature. It is also the natural response to stress, either psychological or physical. Most people have experienced sweaty palms when "put on the spot" or stressed psychologically. As an indication of physical stress, "cold sweat" is helpful in determining the urgency of a problem. If pain is severe or an illness serious, a common effect is a cold sweat. Sweating without other complaints is unusual; as an isolated symptom it is not likely to be serious. In contrast, a cold sweat in a patient complaining of chest pain, abdominal pain, or lightheadedness indicates a need for immediate attention. Remember, however, that aspirin often causes sweating in lowering a fever; sweating associated with the breaking of a fever is not the "cold sweat" referred to here.

Severe pain. Surprisingly enough, severe pain is rarely the symptom which determines that a problem is serious and urgent. Most often it is associated with other symptoms which indicate the nature of the condition; the most obvious example is pain associated with major injury—like a broken leg— which itself clearly requires urgent care. The severity of pain is subjective and depends upon the particular patient; often the magnitude of the pain has been altered by emotional and psychological factors. Nevertheless, severe pain demands urgent medical attention, if for no other reason than to relieve the pain.

Much of the art and science of medicine is directed at the relief of pain, and the use of emergency procedures to secure this relief are justified even if the cause of the pain eventually proves to be inconsequential. However, the patient who frequently complains of severe pain from minor causes is in much the same situation as the boy who cried "wolf"; calls for help will inevitably be taken less and less seriously by the doctor. This situation is a dangerous one, for the patient may have more difficulty in obtaining help when it is most needed.

Work out a procedure for medical emergencies. Develop and test it before an actual emergency arises. If you plan the action you will take ahead of time, you will decrease the likelihood of panic and increase the probability of receiving the proper care quickly.

C
Common Injuries

1 Cuts (Lacerations)

Most cuts affect only the skin and the fatty tissue beneath it. Usually, they heal without permanent damage. However, injury to internal structures such as muscles, tendons, ligaments, blood vessels, or nerves presents the possibility of permanent damage. Your physician can decrease this likelihood.

A cut on the face, chest, abdomen, or back is potentially more serious than one on the extremities. Luckily, most lacerations do occur on the extremities. Cuts on the trunk or face should be examined by a physician unless the injury is very small or extremely shallow. If you see fat protruding from the wound, see the doctor.

You may find it difficult to determine whether major blood vessels, nerves, or arteries have been damaged. Numbness, blood pumping vigorously from the wound, or a tingling or weakness in the affected limb all call for examination by a physician.

Signs of infection—pus oozing from the wound, fever, extensive redness and swelling —will not appear for at least 24 hours. Bacteria need time to grow and multiply. If these signs do appear, a physician must be consulted.

Stitching (suturing) a laceration is a ritual in our society. The only purpose in suturing a wound is to pull the edges together to hasten healing and minimize scarring. If the wound can be held closed without the use of stitches, they are not recommended, as they themselves injure tissue to some extent.

Home Treatment

Cleanse the wound. Soap and water will do, but *be vigorous.* Make sure that no dirt, glass, or other foreign material remains in the wound. This is very important. "Antiseptics" such as mercurochrome or merthiolate are unlikely to help, however, hydrogen peroxide may be used as a cleansing agent. Iodine will kill germs, but is not really needed; if you use iodine, wash the skin afterwards—iodine can burn. (Betadine usually stings less.)

The edges of a clean, minor cut can usually be held together by "butterfly" bandaids or "steri-strips" (preferred)—strips of *sterile* paper tape. Apply either of these bandages so that the edges of the wound join without "rolling under" and without trapping bits of the fatty layer between the edges. Fat protruding from the wound is particularly common in chin lacerations. In a young child who drools, such wounds are often too wet to treat with bandages, so the doctor is usually needed. If the wound cannot be closed without trapping the fat, the laceration needs stitching.

Stitching must take place within eight hours of the injury, because germs begin to grow in the wound and can be trapped under the skin to fester. Thus the chart says "See physician now." Decide immediately whether to see a physician or treat at home. Also refer to Tetanus Shots, Problem 5.

What to Expect at the Doctor's Office

The wound will be thoroughly cleansed, and explored to be sure that no foreign bodies are left in the wound and that blood vessels, nerves, or tendons are undamaged. The physician may use an anesthetic to deaden the area. Be aware of any allergy to lidocaine (Xylocaine) or other local anesthetics; report any possible allergy to the physician. The physician will determine need, if any, for a tetanus shot and decide whether antibiotics are needed (usually not). Lacerations which may require a surgical specialist include those with injury to tendons or major vessels, especially when this damage has occurred in the hand. Facial cuts may also require a surgical specialist if a good cosmetic result appears difficult to obtain.

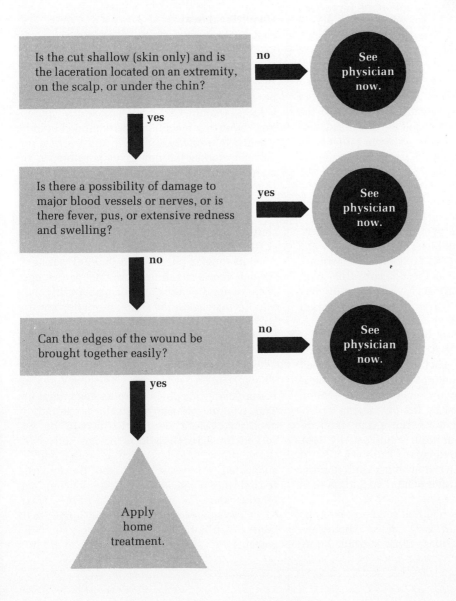

Is the cut shallow (skin only) and is the laceration located on an extremity, on the scalp, or under the chin?

no → See physician now.

yes ↓

Is there a possibility of damage to major blood vessels or nerves, or is there fever, pus, or extensive redness and swelling?

yes → See physician now.

no ↓

Can the edges of the wound be brought together easily?

no → See physician now.

yes ↓

Apply home treatment.

2 Puncture Wounds

Puncture wounds are those caused by nails, pins, tacks and other sharp objects. Usually the only important question is whether a tetanus shot is needed. Consult Tetanus Shots, Problem 5, to determine this. Occasionally punctures do occur in which further medical attention is required.

Most minor puncture wounds are located in the extremities, particularly the feet. If the puncture wound is located on the head, abdomen, or chest a hidden internal injury may have occurred. Unless the wound is obviously minor, see a physician.

Injury to a nerve or to a major blood vessel is rare but can be serious. Injury to an artery may be indicated by blood pumping vigorously from the wound; injury to a nerve usually causes numbness or tingling in the wounded limb, beyond the site of the wound. Major injuries such as these occur rarely with a narrow implement such as a needle; they are more likely with a nail, ice pick, or larger instrument.

To avoid infection, be absolutely sure that nothing has been left in the wound. Sometimes, for example, part of a needle will break off and remain in the foot. If there is any question of a foreign body remaining, the wound should be examined by the physician.

Signs of infection do *not* occur immediately at the time of injury and usually take at least 24 hours to develop. The formation of pus, a fever, or severe swelling and redness are indications that the wound should be seen by a physician.

Many physicians feel that puncture wounds of the hand, if not very minor, should be treated with antibiotics. Once started, infections deep in the hand are difficult to treat and may lead to loss of function. Call the physician for advice if a deep puncture wound of the hand (not the fingers) has occurred.

Home Treatment

Clean the wound to prevent infection. Let it bleed as much as possible to carry foreign material to the outside, since you cannot scrub the inside of a puncture wound. Do *not* apply pressure to stop the bleeding unless there is a large amount of blood loss and a "pumping," squirting bleeding. The wound should be washed thoroughly with soap and warm water and checked as thoroughly as possible for remaining foreign objects. Hydrogen peroxide (dilute to 3%) can be used to cleanse the wound.

Soak the wound in warm water several times a day for four to five days. The object of the soaking is to keep the skin puncture open as long as possible, so that any germs or foreign debris can drain from the open wound. If the wound is allowed to close, an infection may form beneath the skin but not become apparent for several days. Consult Tetanus Shots, Problem 5.

What to Expect at the Doctor's Office

The physician will answer the questions on the opposite chart by history and examination. The wound will be surgically explored, if necessary. More frequently, it will be observed for a reaction to a foreign body over the next few days. If a metallic foreign body is suspected, x-rays may be taken. Be prepared to tell the physician the date of your last tetanus shot; be accurate to within a year. Most physicians will recommend home treatment. Antibiotics will only rarely be suggested.

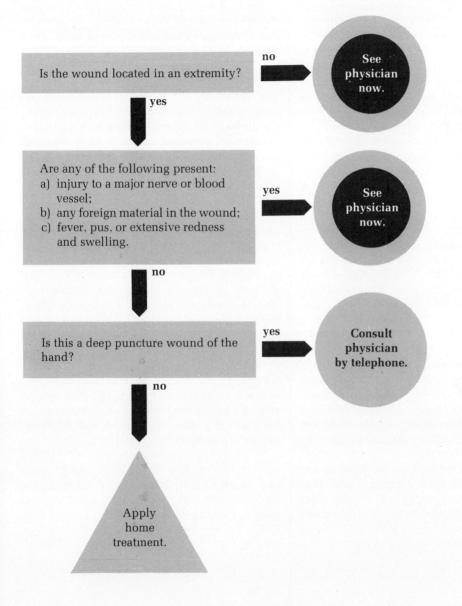

Is the wound located in an extremity?

no → See physician now.

yes ↓

Are any of the following present:
a) injury to a major nerve or blood vessel;
b) any foreign material in the wound;
c) fever, pus, or extensive redness and swelling.

yes → See physician now.

no ↓

Is this a deep puncture wound of the hand?

yes → Consult physician by telephone.

no ↓

Apply home treatment.

3 Animal Bites

The question of rabies is uppermost in the minds of most patients following an animal bite. The main carriers of rabies are wild animals, especially squirrels, skunks, and foxes. Rabies in a pet dog is rare, since most have been immunized at least once. Rabid animals act strangely, attack without provocation, are often thirsty, and may foam at the mouth. Be concerned if your attacker has any of these characteristics.

Any bite by an animal other than a pet dog or cat requires consultation with the physician as to whether or not the use of antirabies vaccine will be required. If the bite is by a dog or a cat, the animal is being reliably observed for sickness by its owner, and its immunizations are up to date, then consultation with the physician may not be required. If the bite has left a wound which might require stitching or other treatment, consult Cuts, Problem 1, or Puncture Wounds, Problem 2. You should also check Tetanus Shots, Problem 5.

Home Treatment

An animal whose immunizations are up to date is, of course, unlikely to have rabies. However, arrange for the animal to be observed for the next 15 days to make sure that it does not develop rabies. Most often, the owners of the animal can be relied upon to observe it. If the owners cannot be trusted, then the animal must be kept for observation by the local public agency charged with that responsibility. Many localities require that animal bites be reported to the health department. If the animal should develop rabies during this time, a very serious situation exists and treatment by a physician must be begun immediately.

For the wound itself, use soap and water. Treat bites as Cuts (see Problem 1) or Puncture Wounds (Problem 2), depending upon their appearance.

What to Expect at the Doctor's Office

The physician must balance the usually remote possibility of exposure to rabies against the hazards of rabies vaccine and antirabies serum. An unprovoked attack by a wild animal, or a bite from an animal which appears to have rabies, may require both the rabies vaccine and the antirabies serum. The extent and location of the wounds also play a part in this decision; severe wounds of the head are the most dangerous.

A bite caused by an animal which has then escaped will often require the use of at least the rabies vaccine. This is one of the most difficult decisions in medicine. Rabies vaccine is administered in 14 to 21 daily injections, which are followed by booster injections 10 to 20 days after the initial series. This vaccine will often cause local skin reactions as well as fever, chills, aches and pain. Severe reactions to the vaccine are rare. The antirabies serum, unfortunately, has a high risk of serious reactions. The serum is given both directly into the wound and by intramuscular injections.

Many physicians give a tetanus shot if you are not "up-to-date" because tetanus bacteria can (rarely) be introduced by an animal bite. Be sure you know when your last tetanus shot was received.

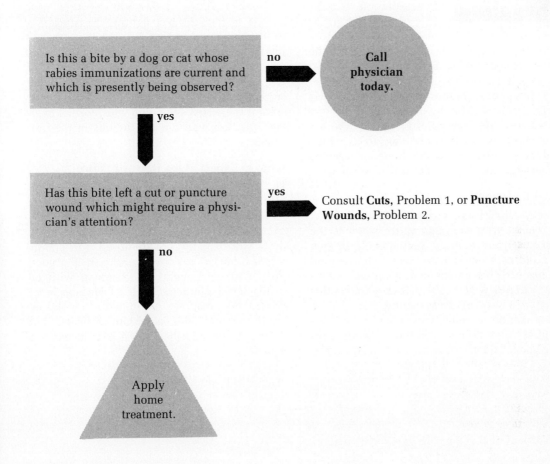

Is this a bite by a dog or cat whose rabies immunizations are current and which is presently being observed?

no → Call physician today.

yes

Has this bite left a cut or puncture wound which might require a physician's attention?

yes → Consult **Cuts,** Problem 1, or **Puncture Wounds,** Problem 2.

no

Apply home treatment.

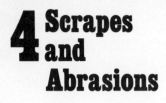 Scrapes and Abrasions

Scrapes and abrasions are shallow. Several layers of the skin may be torn or even totally scraped off, but the wound does not go far beneath the skin. Abrasions are usually caused by falls onto the hands, elbows, or knees, but children and motorcycle riders frequently find ways to get abrasions on just about any part of their bodies.

These injuries are painful. The scrape exposes millions of nerve endings, all of which send pain impulses to the brain. Abrasions are usually much more painful than cuts.

Home Treatment

Remove all dirt and foreign matter. Washing the wound with soap and warm water is the most important step in treatment. Hydrogen peroxide may be used to cleanse the wound but has little advantage over soap and water. Most scrapes will "scab" rather quickly; this is nature's way of dressing the wound. The use of mercurochrome, iodine, and other "antiseptics" may do no harm but certainly does little good. The use of adhesive bandages may be necessary for a wound which continues to ooze blood, but they should be discontinued as soon as possible to allow air and sun to the wound.

Loose skin flaps, if they are not dirty, may be left to help form a natural dressing. If a skin flap is dirty, cut it off carefully with nail scissors. (If it hurts, stop! You're cutting the wrong tissue.) Watch the wound for signs of infection—pus, a fever, or severe swelling or redness, but don't be worried by redness around the edges—this indicates normal healing. Infection will not be obvious in the first 24 hours.

What to Expect at the Doctor's Office

The physician will make sure that the wound is free of dirt and foreign matter. This may sometimes require a local anesthetic to reduce the pain of the cleansing process. Tetanus shots are usually not required for simple scrapes, but, if you are overdue, it is a good chance to get caught up. Dressing with an antibacterial ointment such as Neosporin or Bacitracin sometimes is applied after cleansing the wound. This is seldom of benefit but is frequently done because a patient expects it.

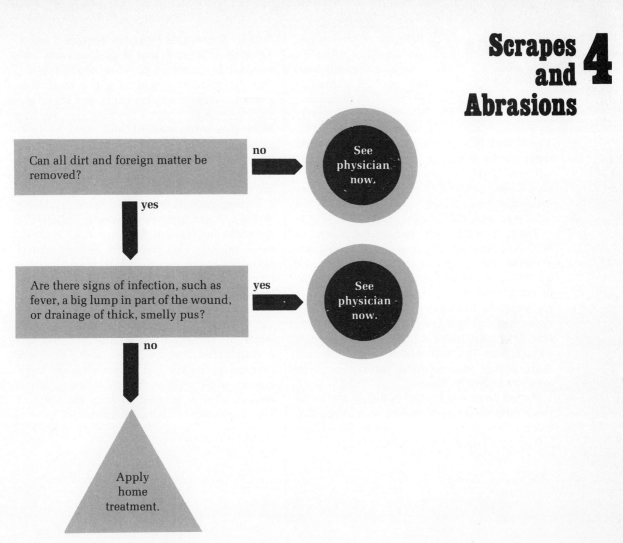

Can all dirt and foreign matter be removed?

no → See physician now.

yes

Are there signs of infection, such as fever, a big lump in part of the wound, or drainage of thick, smelly pus?

yes → See physician now.

no

Apply home treatment.

5 Tetanus Shots

Patients often come to the doctor's office or emergency room simply to "get a tetanus shot." Often the wound is minor and clearly needs only some soap and water. If you don't need the shot, you don't need a doctor in these cases. The chart opposite illustrates the essentials of the current United States Public Health Service recommendations. It can save you and your family several visits to the doctor.

The question of whether or not a wound is "clean and minor" may be troublesome. Wounds caused by sharp, clean objects such as knives or razor blades have less chance of becoming infected than those in which dirt or foreign bodies have penetrated and lodged beneath the skin. Abrasions and minor burns will not result in tetanus. The tetanus germ cannot grow in the presence of air; the skin must be cut or punctured for the germ to reach an airless location.

If you have never had a basic series of three tetanus shots, then you should see the doctor. Sometimes you may require a different kind of tetanus shot if you have not been adequately immunized. This shot is called "tetanus immune globulin," and is used when immunization is not complete and there is a significant risk of tetanus. This shot is more expensive, more painful, and more likely to cause an allergic reaction than is the tetanus "booster." So keep a record of your immunizations in the back of this book and know the dates.

During your first tetanus shots (usually a series of three injections given in childhood), immunity to tetanus develops over a three-week period. This immunity is then slowly lost over many months. After each booster, immunity develops more rapidly and lasts longer. If you have had an initial series of three tetanus injections, immunity will usually last at least ten years after every "booster" injection. Nevertheless, if a wound has left contaminated material beneath the skin, not exposed to the air, and if you have not had a tetanus shot within the past five years, a booster shot is advised to keep the level of your immunity as high as possible.

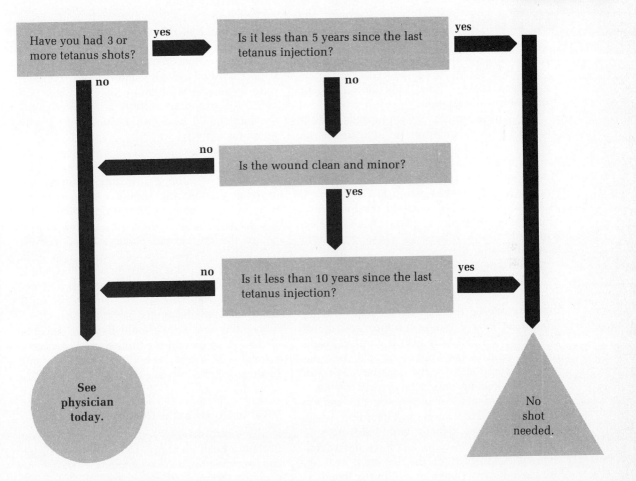

Have you had 3 or more tetanus shots?

yes → Is it less than 5 years since the last tetanus injection?

no

no → Is the wound clean and minor?

yes

no → Is it less than 10 years since the last tetanus injection?

yes

yes

See physician today.

No shot needed.

6 Sprains of Ankle or Knee

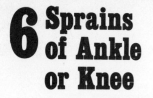

Ligaments are tissues that connect the bones on the opposite sides of a joint to provide stability and create the joint's hinge-like action. When a strong, unusual turn or blow is applied to the joint, ligaments may be stretched (strained), partially torn loose at the ends (sprained), or totally torn (torn ligament).

The typical ankle sprain swells either around the bony bump at the outside of the ankle, or at the top outside of the foot, about two inches forward and below the first location. Sprains are frequently overtreated with unnecessary prolonged rest, casts, and x-rays. A common sense approach to the individual situation is required. Significant knee injuries, especially those related to athletics, should be seen by a physician.

Some basic facts: Usually, an x-ray is only useful to detect a fracture; it does not show injury to soft tissues such as ligaments. Treatment by resting the part is the same (for all conditions except major fracture and major ligament tears). Healing also is similar: swelling and pain in the first 24 to 72 hours, decreasing symptoms for the next ten days, full structural healing only after 6 to 8 weeks.

Torn ligaments are infrequent but seldom heal well without surgery. The joint, while swollen and sore, usually wobbles from side to side, since its stability has been destroyed. Sometimes, instead of the ligament tearing, the portion of the bone to which the ligament is attached tears away instead, creating a fracture. In this case, although the bleeding and bruising beneath the skin may be more pronounced, healing is much like a bad sprain. (A cast may, however, be required.)

Home Treatment

Pain is a warning from your body to stop the activity which caused the pain. Listen to the warning. If it hurts more than a little, don't do it. Don't expect a fully strong joint for six weeks or longer; if you reinjure yourself— start counting again.

Apply an ice pack immediately to decrease the swelling and relieve the pain. Elevate the injured part. Aspirin or acetaminophen (Tylenol) are seldom necessary, but can be used if desired. For ordinary activity, an Ace bandage or an elastic ankle or knee bandage will suffice; if strenuous activity is essential, have the joint taped by a professional—otherwise avoid the activity.

If you have considerable pain when you put weight on the injured part, borrow or rent some crutches for a few days. Adjust the crutches so that the shoulder support is an inch or two short of the armpit. Bear your weight with your hands, *not* in the armpit where the crutch can damage blood vessels and nerves. When you can walk with little discomfort, you can discontinue the crutches. The elastic support may be used during periods of activity for six to eight weeks until the weakened ligaments are fully healed.

Swelling and pain should begin to subside within 48 hours and the limb should be nearly normal within ten days. If your injury is not healing on schedule, see the doctor.

What to Expect at the Doctor's Office

If the chart directs you to the doctor, you probably need an x-ray. Examination will focus on detecting a torn ligament, cartilage, or a major fracture. Standard treatment for uncomplicated cases is the same as home treatment. If much blood is present inside the joint, the physician may drain the blood with a needle. If a ligament is torn, a visit to a surgeon is likely to be recommended. For a major fracture or sprain, a cast may be needed. For many minor fractures, it is not. In severe sprains, the cast is principally to allow performance of necessary normal activities.

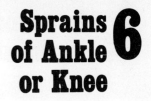

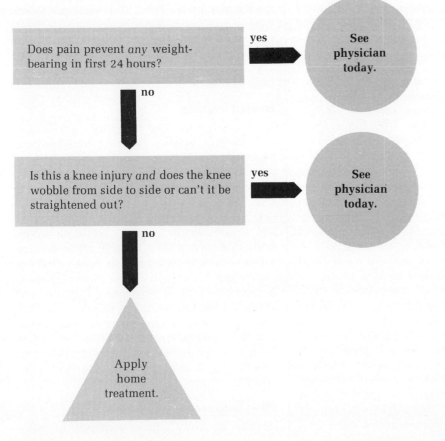

Does pain prevent *any* weight-bearing in first 24 hours?

yes → See physician today.

no

Is this a knee injury *and* does the knee wobble from side to side or can't it be straightened out?

yes → See physician today.

no

Apply home treatment.

7 Is a Bone Broken?

Neither patient nor doctor can always tell by eye whether a bone is broken or not. We have found fractures when we were not expecting them and not found them when we were sure a bone was broken. So you need an x-ray any time there is a reasonable suspicion of a fracture. The chart opposite is a guide to "reasonable suspicion." In the majority of fractures, the bone fragments are already aligned for good healing, thus prompt manipulation of the fragments is not necessary. If the injured part is protected and resting, a delay of several days before casting does no harm. Remember that the cast does not have healing properties, it just keeps the fragments from getting joggled too much during the healing period. Twisting injuries of the knee and ankle are discussed under Sprains, Problem 6.

A fracture can injure near-by nerves and arteries. If the limb is cold, blue, or numb, see the doctor. Fractures of the pelvis or thigh are particularly serious. Check out *all* injuries to these areas with the doctor.

Fortunately these fractures are relatively rare except when great force is involved, as in automobile accidents. In these situations the need for immediate help is usually obvious.

Pallor, sweating, dizziness, and thirst can indicate shock, and immediate attention is needed. For head injuries see Problem 8.

A crooked limb is an obvious reason to check for fracture. The arm bent halfway between elbow and wrist or the leg bent at mid-calf clearly indicates a fracture. Pain which prevents use of the injured limb suggests the need for an x-ray. Soft tissue injuries usually allow some use of the limb, although there are exceptions to this rule.

Although large bruises under the skin may be caused by soft-tissue injuries alone, marked bruising in a limb which may have a fracture means "see the doctor." Common sense tells us that when great force is involved the possibility of a broken bone is increased. The most common example is the automobile accident which often gives us the unwanted opportunity to witness great forces applied to the human body. The child who has fallen twenty feet out of a tree is much more likely to have a broken limb than the child who has stumbled and fallen. The severity of the accident is helpful information, but some bones break with very little provocation.

Home Treatment

Apply ice packs. The immediate application of cold will help to decrease swelling and inflammation. Where a broken bone is suspected, the involved limb should be protected and rested for at least 72 hours. During this time the limb should be cautiously tested to determine persistence of pain on movement and the return of function. The limb which cannot be used at all is more likely to involve a fracture. Any injury which does not show any improvement in pain after 72 hours should be examined by a physician. Minutes and hours are not crucial unless there is misalignment or injury to arteries or nerves. A limb which is adequately protected and rested is likely to have a good outcome even if a fracture is present and casting or splinting is delayed for some time.

What to Expect at the Doctor's Office

Usually, an x-ray will be required. In many offices and emergency rooms, a nurse or physician's assistant will order the x-ray before you are even seen by a physician. In other instances, the physician will examine the injury before ordering the x-ray. In a small number of cases, it is possible to be relatively sure that an x-ray is not needed from the history and physical examination. A crooked limb must be "set." Sometimes this requires general anesthesia. "Pinning" the fragments together surgically so that they will heal well is required for certain fractures.

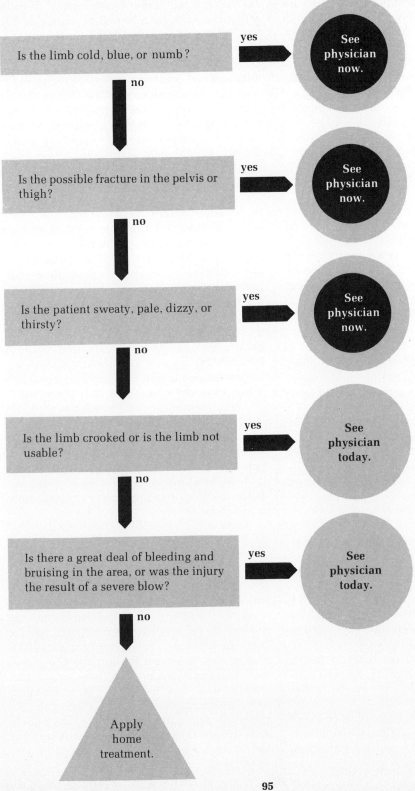

Is the limb cold, blue, or numb? — **yes** → **See physician now.**

no ↓

Is the possible fracture in the pelvis or thigh? — **yes** → **See physician now.**

no ↓

Is the patient sweaty, pale, dizzy, or thirsty? — **yes** → **See physician now.**

no ↓

Is the limb crooked or is the limb not usable? — **yes** → **See physician today.**

no ↓

Is there a great deal of bleeding and bruising in the area, or was the injury the result of a severe blow? — **yes** → **See physician today.**

no ↓

Apply home treatment.

8 Head Injury

All head injuries are potentially serious. Hidden damage can cause major problems long after the injury. Obvious problems are usually brought promptly to a physician's attention, but minor head injuries often result in needless anxiety. Nature has carefully cushioned the valuable contents of the skull. Few minor bumps lead to problems beyond the initial pain. However, careful at-home observation following any head injury is a good idea.

In the following situations, a visit to the physician should not be delayed: bleeding from the ears, eyes, or mouth (may indicate a skull fracture involving a blood vessel); black eyes (same as above—particularly if the bruising surrounds both eyes; unconsciousness (not remembering the injury suggests that unconsciousness was present).

Home Treatment

Ice applied to a bruised area may minimize swelling. Children often develop "goose eggs" anyway. The size of the bump does *not* indicate the severity of the injury.

The observation period is crucial. Bleeding inside the head can cause increased pressure inside the skull over the next 72 hours or more. Check the patient every two hours during the first 24-hour period, every four hours during the second, and every eight hours during the third. Look for the following:

Alertness: Increasing lethargy, unresponsiveness, and *abnormally* deep sleep can precede coma. The seriously affected patient *cannot* be easily roused.

Unequal pupil size: This *can* be caused by increased internal pressure. About 25% of the population have pupils which are unequal all the time—this is normal for them. If pupils become unequal *after* the injury, this is a serious sign.

Severe vomiting: Forceful vomiting may occur and may travel several feet. If significant, repeated vomiting occurs, see the physician.

In the typical minor head injury, a child falls off a table or tree and bangs his or her head. A bump immediately begins to develop. The child remains conscious, although initially stunned. For a few minutes the child is unconsolable and may vomit once or twice over the first couple of hours. Some sleepiness from the excitement may be noted; the child may nap, but is easily aroused. Neither pupil is enlarged and the vomiting ceases shortly. Within eight hours, the child is back to normal except for the tender and often prominent "goose egg."

In a more severe head injury, the child who has increased internal pressure initially has similar symptoms, however, they take hours to develop. Two or more of the danger signs may be present at the same time, with the symptoms of increased pressure manifesting later. The child remains lethargic beyond the post-excitement period and is not easily aroused. A pupil may enlarge. Vomiting is usually violent, repeated and progressive. A critical sign of a serious complication will not be present one minute and gone the next. But, if you have any doubt, call your physician.

Some internal bleeding problems show up even months after the injury. These are called "subdural hematomas" and may cause a chronic headache or personality changes. If you develop such complaints, be sure to mention the head injury to the doctor. This condition is difficult to diagnose, but fortunately is not common.

What to Expect at the Doctor's Office

Don't expect or insist on a skull x-ray. They are seldom useful. There is no treatment for a skull fracture, unless the fragments are pushed in so far that they impinge on the brain or affect a nerve or sense organ. Neck x-rays may, however, be needed. The physician will examine the head, ears, eyes, nose, throat, neck, test the neurological function, and then emphasize the importance of the observation period discussed above. The patient with severe injuries may be hospitalized for the observation period.

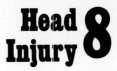

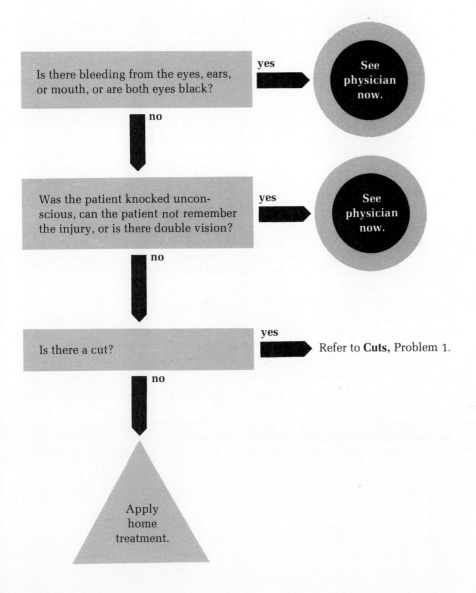

Is there bleeding from the eyes, ears, or mouth, or are both eyes black?

yes → See physician now.

no ↓

Was the patient knocked unconscious, can the patient *not* remember the injury, or is there double vision?

yes → See physician now.

no ↓

Is there a cut?

yes → Refer to **Cuts,** Problem 1.

no ↓

Apply home treatment.

9 Burns

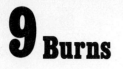

How bad is a burn? Burns are classified as first, second, and third degree, according to the depth of the burn. First degree burns are superficial and cause the skin to turn red. A sunburn is usually a first degree burn. Second degree burns are deeper, and result in splitting of the skin layers or blistering. Scalding with hot water or a very severe sunburn with blisters are common instances of second degree burns. Third degree burns destroy all layers of the skin and extend into the deeper tissues. They are painless because nerve endings have been destroyed. Charring of the burned tissue is usually present.

First degree burns present a problem in pain control but are not a major medical problem. Even when they are extensive, they seldom give rise to lasting problems. Second degree burns are also painful and extensive second-degree burns may cause significant fluid loss. Scarring, however, is usually minimal and infection usually is not a problem. Third degree burns result in scarring and present frequent problems with infection and fluid loss. The more extensive the burn the more difficult these problems.

First degree burns seldom need a doctor's attention. Second degree burns can be treated at home if they are not extensive. Any second degree burn which involves more than 20 or 30 square inches of skin is extensive. In addition, a second-degree burn that involves the face or hands should be seen by a physician; these might result in cosmetic problems or loss of function. All third degree burns should be seen by a physician because these burns lead to scarring and infection, and skin grafts are often needed.

Home Treatment

Apply something cold immediately. This reduces the amount of skin damage done by the burn, and also eases pain. The cold should be applied for at least five minutes and continued until pain is relieved or for one hour, whichever comes first. It may be reapplied if pain returns. Aspirin may be used to reduce pain. Blisters should not be ruptured. If they burst by themselves, as they often do, the overlying skin should be allowed to remain as a "wet dressing." The use of local anesthetic creams or sprays is not recommended as they may slow healing. Also some patients develop irritation or allergy to these drugs. Any burn which continues to be painful for more than 48 hours should be seen by a physician.

What to Expect at the Doctor's Office

The physician will establish the extent and degree of the burn and will determine the need for antibiotics, hospitalization, and skin grafting. An antibacterial ointment and dressing, with frequent changes and checks for infection, will often be recommended for limited third degree burns. Extensive burns may require hospitalization and third degree burns may eventually require skin grafts.

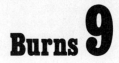

Is this a second degree burn which is:
a) extensive
b) on the face or hands,
or is it a third degree burn?

yes

See
physician
now.

no

Apply
home
treatment.

10 Infected Wounds & Blood Poisoning

"Blood poisoning" is not a current medical term. There is a folk saying that red streaks running up the arm or leg from a wound are "blood poisoning" and that the patient will die when the streaks reach the heart. In fact, such streaks are only inflammation of the lymph channels carrying away the debris from the wound. They will stop when they reach local lymph node in the armpit or groin and do not, by themselves, indicate either infection or blood poisoning.

"Blood poisoning," to a physician, means bacterial infection in the bloodstream, and is termed "septicemia." Fever is a better guide to this rare occurrence. A local wound should only give a very minor temperature elevation unless infected. If you have a fever that you think might be caused by your wound, see your doctor.

An infected wound usually festers beneath the surface of the skin, resulting in pain and swelling. Bacterial infection requires at least a day, and usually two or three days, to develop. Therefore, a late increase in pain or swelling is a legitimate cause for concern. If the festering wound bursts open, pus will drain out. This is good, and the wound will usually heal well. Still, this demonstrates that an infection was present, and the doctor should evaluate the situation unless it is clearly minor.

Why does normal wound healing alarm people so frequently? A few simple facts are missing for most people. First, the body pours out serum into a wound area. Serum is yellowish, clear, and later turns into a "scab." Serum is frequently mistaken for pus, which is thick, cheesy, smelly, and never seen in the first day or so. Second, inflammation around a wound is normal. In order to heal an area, the body must remove the debris and bring in new materials. Thus the edges of a wound will be pink or red, and the wound area may be warm, without an infection. Third, the lymphatic system is actively involved in debris clearance, and pain along lymph channels or in the lymph nodes themselves may be present, without infection.

Home Treatment

Keep a wound clean. If it is unsightly or in a location where it gets dirty easily, bandage it, changing bandages daily; if not, leave it open to the air. Soak and clean it gently with warm water for short periods—three or four times daily to remove debris and keep the scab soft. Don't pick at the scab, let it come loose by itself. Don't be in a hurry. The simplest wound of the face requires 4 to 5 days for healing. The healing period is 7 to 9 days for the chest and arms and 10 to 12 days for the legs. Larger wounds, or those which have gaped open and have to heal across a space, take correspondingly longer to heal. Older people heal more slowly than children.

What to Expect at the Doctor's Office

Examination of the wound and regional lymph nodes. Temperature will be taken. Sometimes, cultures of the blood or of the wound. Sometimes antibiotics are prescribed. If there is a suspicion of bacterial infection then cultures should be taken *before* the antibiotics are given. If a wound is festering it may be drained either with a needle or a scalpel. This procedure is not very painful and actually relieves discomfort. For severe wound infections, hospitalization may be needed.

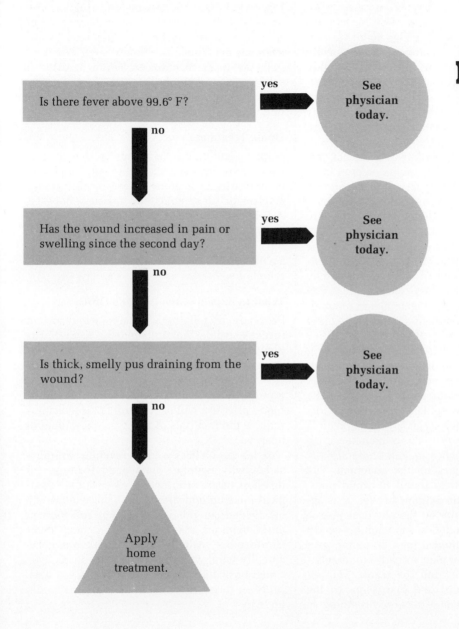

Is there fever above 99.6° F?

yes → **See physician today.**

no ↓

Has the wound increased in pain or swelling since the second day?

yes → **See physician today.**

no ↓

Is thick, smelly pus draining from the wound?

yes → **See physician today.**

no ↓

Apply home treatment.

11 Insect Bites or Stings

Most insect bites are trivial. Nevertheless, they often cause a lot of concern. Insect bites or stings may cause reactions either locally or in the basic body systems. Local reactions may be uncomfortable, but do not pose a serious hazard. In contrast, "systemic" reactions occasionally may be serious and may require emergency treatment.

There are three types of systemic reactions. All of these are rare. The most common is an asthma attack. Here, the patient has difficulty breathing and may have audible wheezing. Hives or skin rashes following insect bites are less serious but indicate that a reaction has occurred and a more severe reaction might occur if the patient is bitten or stung again. Very rarely, fainting or loss of consciousness may occur. If a patient has lost consciousness you must assume that the collapse is due to an allergic reaction. The patient should be taken to an emergency room or to the physician's office at once. If a patient has had any of these reactions in the past, he or she should go immediately to a medical facility if stung or bitten.

Bites from poisonous spiders are rare. The female black widow spider accounts for most of them. This spider is glossy black with a body approximately ½ inch in diameter, a leg span of about 2 inches, and a characteristic red "hour-glass" mark on the abdomen. The black widow spider is found in wood piles, sheds, basements, or outdoor privies. It is aggressive and may bite on the slightest provocation. The bite produces a momentary sharp pain at the site, followed by a cramping pain within the hour. The pain spreads and may involve all extremities and the trunk. The abdomen becomes hard and board-like as the waves of pain become severe. Breathing is difficult and accompanied by grunting. There may be nausea, vomiting, headaches, sweating, twitching, and shaking, and tingling sensations of the hand. The bite itself may not be prominent and may be overshadowed by the systemic reaction.

If the local reaction to a bite or sting is severe or an ulcer is developing at the site, then a physician should be consulted by phone.

Home Treatment

Apply something cold promptly. Ice or cold packs may be used. Delay in application of cold results in a more severe local reaction. Aspirin or other pain relievers may be used. Antihistamines, such as Benadryl, do not decrease the reaction very much; they may relieve the itching somewhat. If the reaction is severe, the physician may be consulted by telephone.

What to Expect at the Doctor's Office

Be ready to tell the physician what sort of insect or spider has inflicted the wound. The physician will search for signs of systemic reaction. If a systemic reaction is present, adrenalin by injection is usually necessary. Rarely, measures to support breathing or blood pressure will be needed; these measures require the facilities of an emergency room or hospital.

If the problem is a local reaction, the physician will examine the wound for signs of death of tissue or infection. Occasionally, surgical incision and drainage of the wound will be needed. In other cases, pain relievers or antihistamines may make the patient more comfortable. Adrenalin injections are occasionally employed for very severe local reactions. Basically, these measures cause a local problem to go away about as fast as it would anyway.

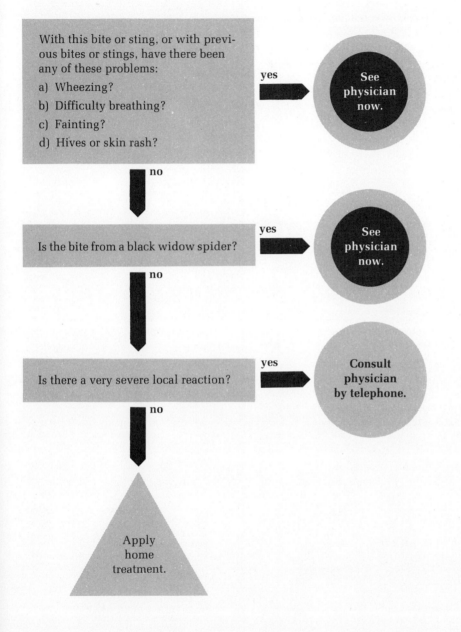

With this bite or sting, or with previous bites or stings, have there been any of these problems:

a) Wheezing?
b) Difficulty breathing?
c) Fainting?
d) Hives or skin rash?

yes → **See physician now.**

no

Is the bite from a black widow spider?

yes → **See physician now.**

no

Is there a very severe local reaction?

yes → **Consult physician by telephone.**

no

Apply home treatment.

D
Poisons

12 Oral Poisoning

Although poisons may be inhaled or absorbed through the skin, for the most part they are swallowed. The term "ingestion" refers to oral poisoning, and is often used as a euphemism for "suicide attempt."

Most poisonings can be prevented. Children almost always swallow poison accidentally. Keep harmful substances, such as prescribed medications, insecticides, caustic cleansers, and organic solvents, out of the reach of little hands. The most notorious are strong alkali solutions, used as drain cleaners (Drano), which will destroy any tissue with which it comes in contact.

Treatment must be prompt to be effective, but, while speed is important, accurate identification of the ingested substance is equally so. *Don't Panic*. Call the doctor or poison control center immediately and get advice on what to do. Attempt to identify the substance without causing undue delay; if you can't, bring the container to the emergency room with you or leave someone behind to identify the substance and telephone in the information. Life-support measures take precedence in the case of the unconscious victim, but the ingested substance must be identified before proper therapy can be employed.

Suicide attempts cause most significant medication overdoses. Any suicide attempt is an indication that psychiatric help is needed. Such help is not optional, even if the patient has "recovered" and is in no immediate danger. Most successful suicides are preceded by unsuccessful attempts.

Home Treatment

All cases of poisoning should be reported to a physician; home treatment in this case is "first-aid" and should always be followed by a call to the poison control center or doctor. If the patient is conscious and alert, and the ingredients swallowed are known, there are two types of treatment: those in which vomiting should be induced, and those in which it should not. Usually, vomiting is desirable, but not if the poison contained strong acids, alkalis, or petroleum products. These substances can destroy the gullet or inflame the lungs as they are vomited. Neutralize them with milk while contacting the physician. If you don't have milk give some water or some milk of magnesia.

With most poisons, emptying the stomach will remove unabsorbed poison. Vomiting is more effective and safer than the "stomach pump" and can be induced by a parent or by the patient. In an alert patient vomiting is safe unless an acid, alkali, or petroleum product was ingested. Vomiting can be achieved immediately by stimulating the back of the throat with a finger (don't be squeamish!), or by two to four teaspoonfuls of syrup of ipecac, followed by as much liquid as the child can drink. The exact dosage is not critical, since it won't be staying down, anyway. Vomiting follows usually within ten minutes but, since time is important, the finger is quicker. Or you can try both. Collect the vomitus so that it may be examined by the physician, if necessary.

Before, after, or during first-aid, contact a physician. Many communities have established "poison control centers" to identify poisons and give advice. Poison control centers are often located in emergency rooms. Find out if such a center exists in your community and, if so, record the telephone number both on the chart and in the front of this book. Quick first-aid and fast professional advice are your best chance to avoid a tragedy.

What to Expect at the Doctor's Office

Significant poisoning is best managed at the emergency room. An unconscious patient will be admitted to the hospital. Treatment of the conscious patient is dependent upon the particular poison and whether vomiting has been successfully achieved. Ingestion of strong alkalis, strong acids, and petroleum products usually will require admission to the hospital. Otherwise, the stomach will be evacuated by vomiting or by the use of a stomach pump. In patients not admitted to the hospital, observation at home is important.

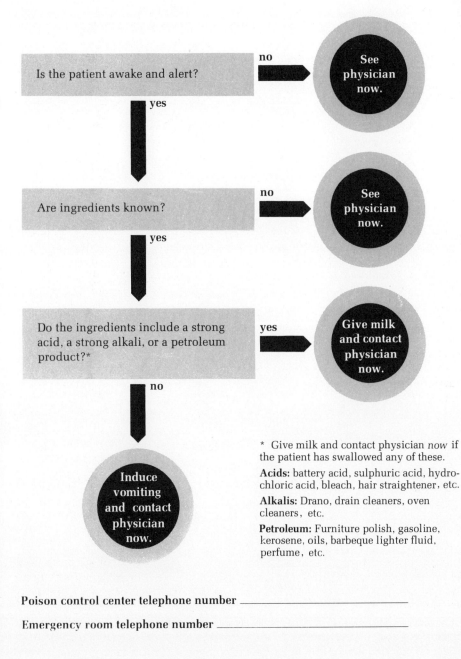

Is the patient awake and alert? — **no** → See physician now.

↓ **yes**

Are ingredients known? — **no** → See physician now.

↓ **yes**

Do the ingredients include a strong acid, a strong alkali, or a petroleum product?* — **yes** → Give milk and contact physician now.

↓ **no**

Induce vomiting and contact physician now.

* Give milk and contact physician *now* if the patient has swallowed any of these.

Acids: battery acid, sulphuric acid, hydrochloric acid, bleach, hair straightener, etc.

Alkalis: Drano, drain cleaners, oven cleaners, etc.

Petroleum: Furniture polish, gasoline, kerosene, oils, barbeque lighter fluid, perfume, etc.

Poison control center telephone number _____

Emergency room telephone number _____

E

The Ears, Nose, and Throat

IS IT A VIRUS, BACTERIA, OR AN ALLERGY?

The following sections discuss upper respiratory problems, including colds and "flu," sore throats, ear pain or stuffiness, runny nose, cough, hoarseness, swollen glands, nosebleeds. A central question is important to each of these complaints: is it caused by a virus, or bacteria, or an allergic reaction? In general, only for bacterial infection does the doctor have more effective treatment than is available at home. The fact to remember is: viral infections and allergies do *not* improve with treatment by penicillin or other antibiotics. To demand a "penicillin shot" for a cold or allergy is to ask for a drug reaction, risk a more serious "super-infection," and to waste time and money. Among common problems well treated at home are:

- the common cold—often termed "viral URI (Upper Respiratory Infection)" by doctors.

- The flu when uncomplicated.

- Hayfever.

- Mononucleosis—infectious mononucleosis or "mono."

Medical treatment *is* commonly required for:

- Strep throat.

- Ear infection.

How can you tell these conditions apart? Table 2 and the charts for the following problems will usually suffice. Here are some brief descriptions.

Viral syndromes—Viruses usually involve several portions of the body and cause many different symptoms. Three basic patterns (or syndromes) are common in viral illnesses:

Viral URI—This is the "common cold." It includes some combination of the following: sore throat, runny nose, stuffy or congested ears, hoarseness, swollen glands, and fever. One symptom usually precedes the others and another (usually hoarseness or cough) may remain after the others have disappeared.

The flu—Fever may be quite high. Headache can be excruciating, muscle aches and pain (especially low back and eye muscles) are equally troublesome.

Viral gastroenteritis—This is the "stomach flu" with nausea, vomiting, diarrhea and crampy abdominal pain. It may be incapacitating and can mimic a variety of other more serious conditions including appendicitis.

Overlap between these three syndromes is not unusual. Your illness may sometimes have features of each.

Hayfever—The seasonal runny nose and itchy eyes are well-known. Patients themselves usually diagnose this condition accurately. As with viruses, this

111

Is it a virus,
bacteria,
or an allergy?

disorder is treated simply to relieve symptoms; given enough time the condition runs its course without doing any permanent harm. Allergies tend to recur whenever the pollen or other allergic substance is encountered.

Strep throat—Bacterial infections tend to localize at a single point. Involvement of the respiratory tract by strep is usually limited to the throat. However, symptoms outside the respiratory tract can occur, most commonly fever and swollen lymph glands (from draining the infected material) in the neck. The rash of scarlet fever sometimes may help to distinguish a streptococcal (strep) from a viral infection. In children, abdominal pain may be associated with a strep throat. This disorder must be diagnosed and treated, since serious heart and kidney complications can follow if adequate antibiotic therapy is not given.

Other conditions—Factors other than diseases may cause or contribute to upper respiratory symptoms. Smoking accounts for a large number of coughs and sore throats. Public pollution (smog) can produce the same problems. Tumor and other frightening conditions account for only a very small number. Complaints lasting beyond two weeks without one of the common diseases as the obvious cause are not alarming, but should be investigated on a routine basis by the doctor.

TABLE 2
IS IT A VIRUS, BACTERIA, OR AN ALLERGY?

	Virus	Bacteria	Allergy
Runny nose?	Often	Rare	Often
Aching muscles?	Usual	Rare	No
Headache?	Often	Rare	No
Dizzy?	Often	Rare	Rare
Fever?	Often	Often	No
Cough?	Often	Sometimes	Rare
Dry cough?	Often	Rare	Sometimes
Raising sputum?	Rare	Often	Rare
Hoarseness?	Often	Rare	Rare
Recurs at a particular season?	No	No	Often
A single complaint present? (sore throat, earache, sinus pain, cough)	Unusual	Usual	Unusual
Do antibiotics help?	No	Yes	No
Can the doctor help?	Seldom	Yes	Sometimes

Remember, viral infections and allergies *do not* improve with treatment by penicillin or other antibiotics.

13 Colds & Flu

If you have a runny nose, aches and shakes, and are losing your voice while those around you are losing theirs, you undoubtedly have the local bug, the common cold. Seldom is there any doubt. Your misery drives you to seek succor and sympathy. There isn't any. Look at the chart on the facing page. If your problem isn't persistent, isn't associated with unusual symptoms, and isn't settling into a single location such as the throat, ears, or sinuses, you need patience and home treatment.

How long will it last? Ask your friends. Each of the many viruses which cause upper respiratory symptoms has its own incubation period, group of symptoms, and duration. Find out what is going around, there is a good chance that you have the same problem. For more information on viral infections, read "Is it a virus, bacteria or an allergy?"

Home Treatment

"Take two aspirin and call me in the morning." This familiar phrase does *not* mean neglect or lack of sympathy for your problem. Aspirin is the best available medicine for the fever and muscular aches of the common cold. For adults, two five-grain aspirin tablets every four hours is standard treatment. The fever, aches, and prostration are most pronounced in the afternoon and evening; be particularly sure to take the aspirin regularly over this period. If you have trouble tolerating aspirin, use acetaminophen (Tylenol) in the same dose. If you like to spend money, buy a well-known brand-name aspirin or a patent cold formula. But remember, the important ingredient that "doctors recommend most" is aspirin; check labels for equivalent dosage.

"Drink a lot of liquid." This is insurance. The body requires more fluid if you have a fever. Be sure you get enough. Fluids help keep the mucus more liquid, and help prevent complications such as bronchitis and ear infection. A vaporizer (particularly in the winter if you have forced-air heat) will help liquefy secretions.

"Rest." This is gratuitous. If you don't have fever and want to work, go ahead. It won't prolong your illness, and everybody at the office was exposed during the incubation period, before you had symptoms, anyway.

A word for chicken soup: Dizziness when standing up is common with colds, and is helped by drinking salty liquids. Bouillon and chicken soup are excellent.

If symptoms persist beyond two weeks, then see the doctor.

What to Expect at the Doctor's Office

In general, lack of enthusiasm. "For this I spent four years in medical school?" In a busy office you take up valuable time and possibly expose patients with severe lung problems to a virus they can ill tolerate.

The physician will examine nose, throat, and ears, and listen to your lungs. If your throat looks raw, a culture may be taken. You will get the advice above. Perhaps you will be given an antihistamine which will make you sleepier than the ones you can get yourself at the drugstore, or one of a group of combination "cold" compounds available by prescription only. These have similar ingredients to medications available "over-the-counter" and will not shorten the illness.

For an uncomplicated cold, you should not receive an injection or an oral antibiotic. These will not help and have potential for harm.

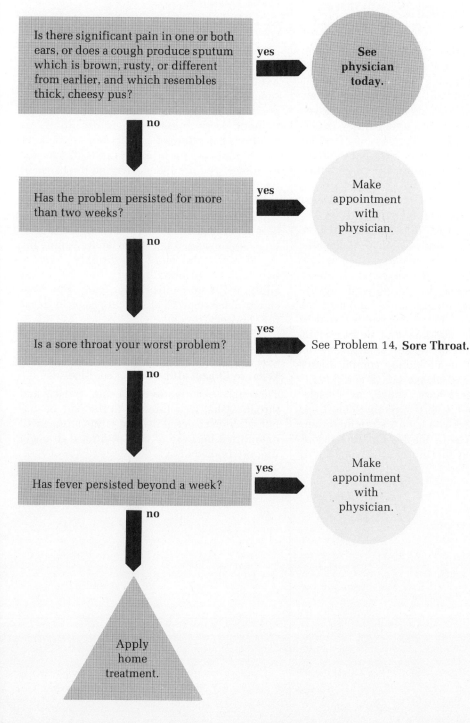

Is there significant pain in one or both ears, or does a cough produce sputum which is brown, rusty, or different from earlier, and which resembles thick, cheesy pus?

yes → **See physician today.**

no ↓

Has the problem persisted for more than two weeks?

yes → Make appointment with physician.

no ↓

Is a sore throat your worst problem?

yes → See Problem 14, **Sore Throat.**

no ↓

Has fever persisted beyond a week?

yes → Make appointment with physician.

no ↓

Apply home treatment.

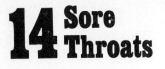 Sore Throats

"Strep throat" is a sore throat caused by the streptococcus bacteria and can lead to complications of rheumatic fever or kidney disease. A throat culture is the most accurate method for determining if the problem is strep. An increasing number of physicians are enabling their patients to get throat cultures without seeing the physician first. We applaud and encourage this movement since it eliminates unnecessary office visits and saves money. The cost of an office visit *and* throat culture may be twenty dollars or more, while the charge for a throat culture alone may be two to five dollars. Request a throat culture without a physician examination; the office nurse can take the culture.

If you have been exposed to strep, if you have a rash, or if you have had rheumatic fever or kidney disease in the past, it is important for you to see the physician. In these cases, antibiotics may be started while awaiting the culture results. Because immunity develops after several infections, strep throat is most common in children and decreases in frequency with advancing age. It is unusual to see rheumatic fever or kidney complications for the first time after age 25. If you have a runny nose, hoarseness, cough, or muscle aches and pains, it is very unlikely to be strep. Most of the time, if you have a strep infection, pus will be visible in the back of the throat when you look in the throat with good light.

If it's not strep throat, home treatment is as effective as any. For more information, read "Is it a virus, bacteria or an allergy?"

Home Treatment

Antibiotics are not effective against viruses, allergies, or smoking irritation. They are expensive, require a prescription, have potential for dangerous allergic reaction, and should not be used unless the physician strongly suspects strep throat or a throat culture is positive for strep. Symptomatic treatment without prescription drugs is essentially as good as that afforded by the more expensive and harder-to-obtain preparations. If you are a smoker, you are likely carrying the cause of your sore throat in your pocket.

Salt water gargles (½ teaspoon salt in a cup of warm water) and throat lozenges may help relieve pain. A cool room, high fluid intake, and a vaporizer will assist in keeping the throat moist and more comfortable. Aspirin, two tablets (10 grains) every four hours for adults will help control fever, pain, and associated aches. See Chapter 7 for aspirin doses for children.

If the sore throat persists for more than three weeks, see the doctor.

What to Expect at the Doctor's Office

Thorough examination of ears, nose, and throat. Usually, a throat culture will be obtained. In occasional instances the culture will be omitted because of cost or a need to begin therapy immediately.

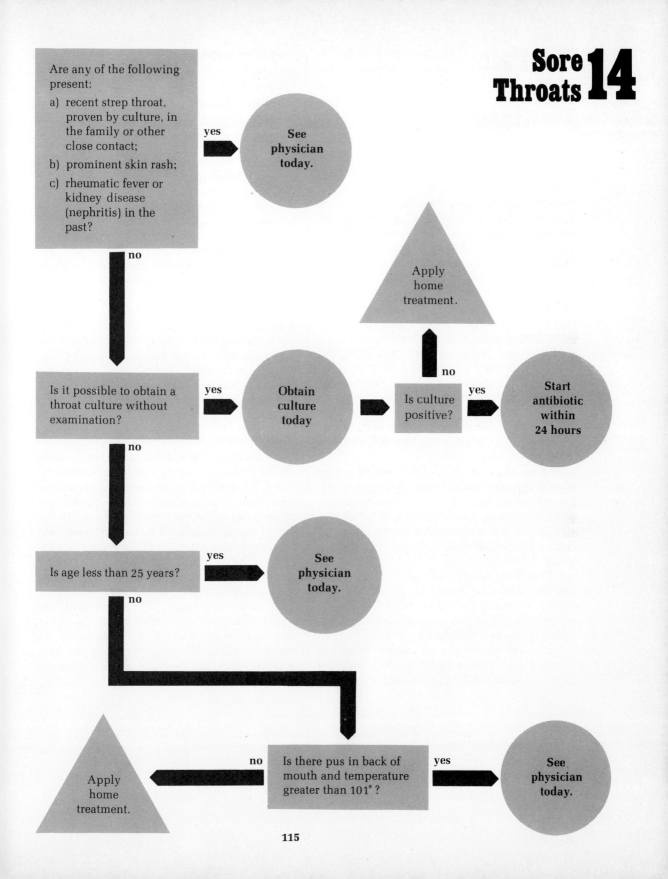

Are any of the following present:

a) recent strep throat, proven by culture, in the family or other close contact;

b) prominent skin rash;

c) rheumatic fever or kidney disease (nephritis) in the past?

yes → **See physician today.**

no ↓

Sore Throats 14

Is it possible to obtain a throat culture without examination?

yes → **Obtain culture today** → Is culture positive? → yes → **Start antibiotic within 24 hours**

no ↑ → **Apply home treatment.**

no ↓

Is age less than 25 years?

yes → **See physician today.**

no ↓

Apply home treatment. ← no ← Is there pus in back of mouth and temperature greater than 101°? → yes → **See physician today.**

115

15 Ear Pain and/or Stuffiness

A severe earache is usually due to a bacterial infection in the middle ear and should be treated with antibiotics. The chart is very, very simple. If it hurts very much, see the doctor. If the passage between the middle ear and the nose (Eustachian tube) is open, then middle ear infection is very rare, because invading bacteria are carried through the tube on a layer of moving mucus and swallowed. Therefore, most middle ear infections follow a blockage of the Eustachian tube by a cold or allergy. An infection may not occur immediately, so that a blocked Eustachian tube may cause fluid to collect behind the ear drum. This causes a stuffy or blocked sensation. After the Eustachian tube is clear, relief is prompt.

Middle ear infection requires antibiotic therapy and many physicians give antibiotics for fluid collected behind the ear to prevent infection. If significant ear pain is present, or if a child cries and holds the ear, see the physician—before the child's bedtime if possible. You, the child, and the physician will all sleep better.

The ear canal outside of the eardrum may also be inflamed or irritated. This type of inflammation is not as severe and does not threaten hearing. In the winter, it is usually allergic. In the summer, "swimmer's ear" is more common. External ear canal irritation is characterized by itching or discharge from the ear. Treatment is usually local. If pain is present, the physician should be consulted. Discharge occurring just after sudden relief of ear pain is not due to external ear infection; it may indicate a perforated ear drum.

Inner ear problems can cause dizziness (vertigo) and trouble with balance. They require the attention of a physician.

Home Treatment

Moisture and humidity are important to keep the mucus thin. Use a vaporizer if you have one. Curious maneuvers (such as hopping up and down in a steamy shower while shaking the head and swallowing) are sometimes dramatically successful in clearing out mucus.

Aspirin or acetaminophen (Tylenol) will provide partial pain relief. See Chapter 7 for doses for children.

Antihistamines and decongestants are used to decrease the amount of nasal secretion and to shrink the mucus membranes. Some common over-the-counter preparations are Contac, Sudafed, Allerest, and Sinutab. Fluid in the ear will often respond to home treatment alone.

External inflammation may be eased by a drop of mineral oil in the ear canal. Do not use a cotton plug for the canal, and do not put objects such as Q-tips and hairpins deep into the ear canal. Place nothing smaller than the patient's elbow into the ear canal.

If symptoms continue beyond two weeks, see the doctor.

What to Expect at the Doctor's Office

Examination of ears, nose, and throat. Antibiotic therapy (usually penicillin or ampicillin) for a period of at least 5 days will be prescribed if the physician notes inflammation of the eardrum or the presence of fluid in the ear. In recurrent infections, the physician may puncture the eardrum or place small tubes through the eardrum. These procedures sound painful and dangerous, but are actually simple, safe, relieve pain, and protect hearing.

If antibiotics have been prescribed, be sure to continue supportive home treatment also. Antibiotics require an average of 24 hours to relieve the pain by killing the bacteria. Keeping the Eustachian tubes clear of mucus will bring faster relief.

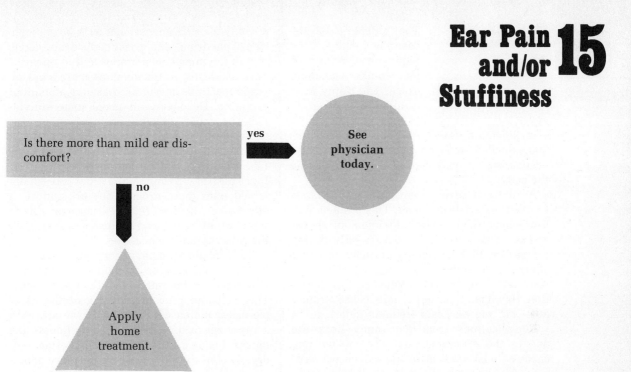

Is there more than mild ear discomfort?

yes → See physician today.

no → Apply home treatment.

16 Runny Nose

The hallmark of the common cold is the runny nose. Allergy is the other common cause. The runny nose is intended by nature to help the body fight virus infection. Nasal secretions contain antibodies which act against viruses. The profuse outpouring of fluid carries the virus outside the body.

A runny nose is often caused by pollens or other materials in the air. This problem will last longer than a viral infection, often for weeks or months, but it occurs only during the season that the pollen particles or other allergens are in the air. Hence, nicknames like "hay fever" have been applied to this condition. Hay itself does not usually cause a runny nose, but ragweed is a frequent culprit.

Complications from the runny nose are due to the excess mucus. The mucus may cause a "post-nasal drip" and cough which is most prominent at night. A great many substances, including house dusts and animal danders, can cause this problem. The mucus drip may plug the Eustachian tube between the nasal passages and the ear, resulting in ear infection and pain. It may plug the sinus passages, resulting in secondary sinus infection and sinus pain. For more information read "Is it a virus, bacteria, or an allergy?"

Home Treatment

Two major types of drugs are used to control a runny nose. Decongestants such as epinephrine, ephedrine, and pseudoephedrine act to shrink the mucus membranes and to open the nasal passages. Antihistamines act to block allergic reactions and to decrease the amount of secretion. Decongestants make some individuals "nervous," and antihistamines may cause drowsiness. Many "cold preparations" available over the counter (Contac, Allerest, Sinutab, Sinarest) contain mixtures of the two types of drugs. Symptomatic relief is often obtained with these drugs. They are almost as effective as the prescription drugs available to treat "runny nose," and are also less toxic than the prescription medications.

Complications such as ear and sinus infection often may be prevented by ensuring that mucus is thin rather than thick and sticky. This helps to prevent plugging of the nasal passages. Increased humidity in the air, with a vaporizer or humidifier, helps to liquefy the mucus. Inside a house, heated air is often very dry. Cooler air contains more moisture and is preferable.

If symptoms persist beyond three weeks, see the doctor.

What to Expect at the Doctor's Office

A thorough examination of nose, ears, throat. A check for tenderness over the sinuses. Temperature. Examination of other areas with associated symptoms. Do not expect antibiotics, such as penicillin, to be prescribed for routine runny-nose symptoms. Antibiotics are not effective against virus or allergy.

Is there a rusty, green, or smelly drainage?

yes → **See physician today.**

no ↓

Apply home treatment.

17 Cough

The cough reflex is one of the body's best "defense mechanisms." Irritation or obstruction in the breathing tubes triggers this reflex, and the violent rush of air helps clear material from the breathing tubes. If abnormal material, such as pus, is being expelled from the body by coughing, then the cough is desirable. Such a cough is termed "productive," and should usually not be suppressed by medication.

Often, a minor irritation or a healing area in a breathing tube will start the cough reflex even though there is no material other than the normal mucus to be expelled. At other times, mucus from the nasal passages will drain into the breathing tubes at night (post-nasal drip) and initiate the cough reflex. Such coughs are not beneficial and may be symptomatically relieved.

The bronchi have another defense mechanism which can take the place of the cough in removing small amounts of pus and other abnormal materials. Small moving hairs transport foreign particles in the mucus to the throat, where they are swallowed. The mucus traps the particle, the hairs move it out. For this mechanism to work, the mucus must be thin rather than thick, and the cells which operate the moving hairs must not be injured by inhaled cigarette smoke or other toxins. For more information on coughs, read "Is it a virus, bacteria or an allergy?"

Home Treatment

The mucus in the breathing tubes may be made thinner and less sticky by several means. Increased humidity in the air will help. A vaporizer and a steamy shower are two ways to increase the humidity of the air. In the severe "croup" cough of small children, high humidity is absolutely essential. Drinking large quantities of fluids is helpful for cough, particularly if a fever has dried out (dehydrated) the body. Glycerol guaiacolate (Robitussin or 2G) is available over-the-counter and helps to liquefy the secretions. The liberal use of such common home substances as pepper and garlic also liquefies the secretions and may help.

Decongestants (such as Contac, Allerest, or Sinutab) may help if a post-nasal drip is causing the cough. Otherwise, avoid drugs which contain antihistamines because they tend to dry the secretions and make them thicker.

Various cough preparations available over-the-counter will afford relief from a bothersome cough. Dry, tickling coughs are often relieved by cough lozenges or sucking on hard candy. Dextromethorphan (Romilar) is an effective cough suppressant, available over-the-counter. Adults may require up to twice the dosage recommended in the package instructions. Do not exceed this amount; neither dextromethorphan nor codeine will completely eliminate most coughs at any dosage, and side effects of drowsiness or constipation can occur.

What to Expect at the Doctor's Office

Examination of the throat and chest. Temperature. Blood count and chest x-ray in some instances. Do not expect antibiotics to be prescribed for a routine viral or allergic cough; they do not help.

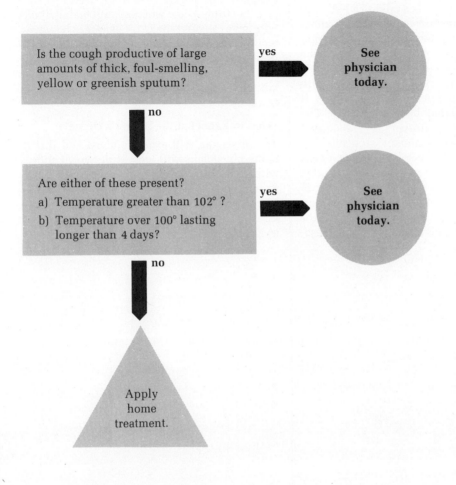

Cough **17**

Is the cough productive of large amounts of thick, foul-smelling, yellow or greenish sputum?

yes → **See physician today.**

no

Are either of these present?
a) Temperature greater than 102°?
b) Temperature over 100° lasting longer than 4 days?

yes → **See physician today.**

no

Apply home treatment.

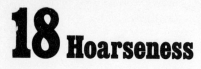18 Hoarseness

Hoarseness is usually caused by irritation of the vocal chords. The most common cause is a cold. As with any symptom of an upper respiratory tract infection, hoarseness may linger after other symptoms disappear. When hoarseness is mild the most common cause is cigarette smoke. If persistent hoarseness is *not* associated with either a viral infection or with smoking, it should be investigated by a physician. The length of the wait is controversial. We suggest one month. If you are a smoker, stop smoking and wait one month. Persistent hoarseness has many causes; the most common are cysts or polyps on the vocal chords. Yes, cancer is also a cause, but is relatively rare. In children, especially, yelling or screaming for a prolonged time is a frequent cause of hoarseness.

Home Treatment

Hoarseness is very resistant to any sort of therapy. Nature must heal the inflamed area. Humidifying the air with a vaporizer or simply "wetting your whistle" by taking fluids will give some relief. In general, however, wait for healing to occur after the viral infection has passed or after the irritation from smoking has ceased. Rest the vocal chords by talking as little as possible and shouting not at all.

What to Expect at the Doctor's Office

The physician will examine chest and throat. Some physicians will look at the vocal chords with the aid of a small mirror. Occasionally, an ear, nose, and throat (ENT) specialist may be consulted for further examinations. A chest x-ray may be ordered, especially if the patient is a smoker.

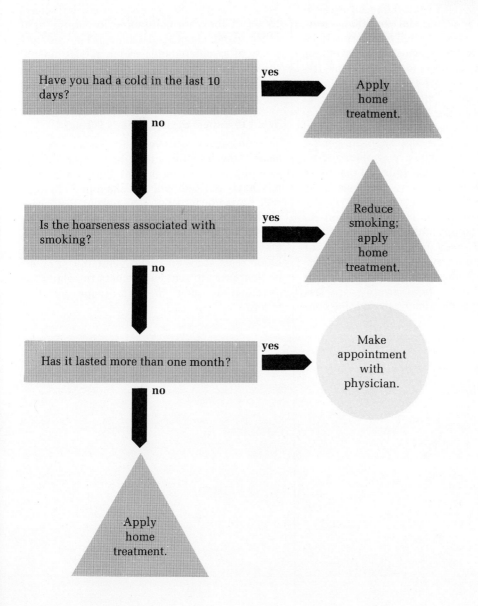

Have you had a cold in the last 10 days?

yes → Apply home treatment.

no ↓

Is the hoarseness associated with smoking?

yes → Reduce smoking; apply home treatment.

no ↓

Has it lasted more than one month?

yes → Make appointment with physician.

no ↓

Apply home treatment.

19 Swollen Glands

Lymph glands are part of the body's defense against infection. They may become swollen even if the infection is trivial or inapparent. Usually you can identify the infection that is causing the swelling. The familiar swollen glands in the neck frequently accompany sore throats or ear infections. Swelling of a gland simply means that it is taking part in the fight against the infection. Glands in the groin are enlarged when there is infection in the legs or in the genital region. Often these glands are swollen and no obvious infection can be found. Sometimes the basic problem may be so trivial as to be overlooked (as with athlete's foot).

Swollen glands themselves require no investigation or therapy unless they persist for several weeks. Glands in the front and side of the neck, or in the groin, are seldom serious. Swollen glands in the back of the neck, above the collarbone, or in both armpits are less common and the physician should be consulted if the swelling persists for more than three weeks.

Home Treatment

Merely observe the glands over several weeks to see if they are continuing to enlarge or if other glands become swollen. The vast majority of swollen glands which persist beyond three weeks are not serious, but a physician should be consulted if the glands show no tendency to become smaller.

What to Expect at the Doctor's Office

The physician will examine the glands and search for infections or other causes of the swelling. Other glands that the patient may not have noticed will be examined. Inquiry will be made into fever or weight loss associated with the swelling of the glands. The physician may decide to simply observe the glands for a period of time, or may decide that blood tests are indicated. Eventually, it might be necessary to remove (biopsy) the gland for examination under the microscope, but this is rare.

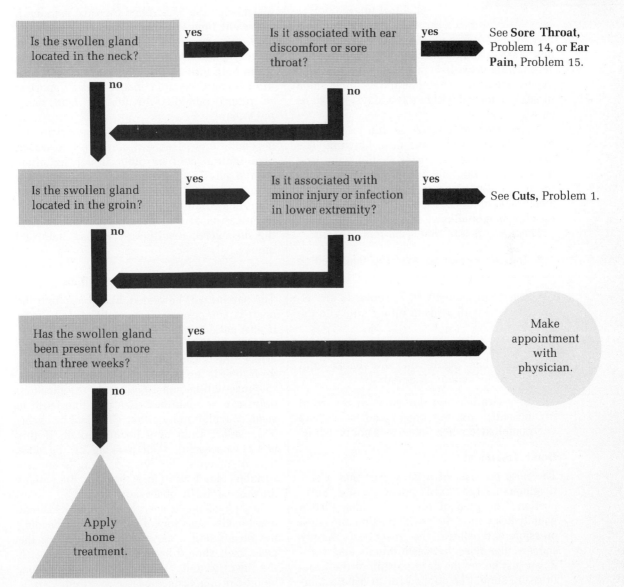

Is the swollen gland located in the neck? — **yes** → Is it associated with ear discomfort or sore throat? — **yes** → See **Sore Throat,** Problem 14, or **Ear Pain,** Problem 15.

no

no

Is the swollen gland located in the groin? — **yes** → Is it associated with minor injury or infection in lower extremity? — **yes** → See **Cuts,** Problem 1.

no

no

Has the swollen gland been present for more than three weeks? — **yes** → Make appointment with physician.

no

Apply home treatment.

20 Nosebleeds

The blood vessels within the nose lie very near the surface and bleeding may occur with the slightest injury.

Medical opinion is divided as to whether nosebleeds can be caused by high blood pressure. Patients with high blood pressure who experience nosebleeds should have their blood pressure checked within a few days, just to be sure.

Nosebleeds are frequently due to irritation by a virus or to vigorous nose blowing. The main problem in this case is the cold, and treatment of the cold symptoms will reduce the probability of a nosebleed. If the mucous membrane of the nose is dry, cracking and bleeding is more likely.

These key points should be remembered:

- You can almost always stop the bleeding yourself;

- The great majority of nosebleeds are associated with colds or minor injury to the nose.

- Treatment such as packing the nose with gauze has significant drawbacks and should be avoided if possible;

- Investigation into the cause of recurrent nosebleeds is not urgent and is best accomplished when the nose is *not* bleeding.

Home Treatment

The nose consists of a bony part and a cartilaginous part; a "hard" portion and a "soft" portion. The area of the nose which bleeds usually lies within the "soft" portion and compression will control the nosebleed. Simply squeeze the nose between thumb and forefinger just below the hard portion of the nose. Pressure should be applied for at least 5 minutes. The patient should be seated with his or her head back and should not lie down. Cold compresses or ice applied across the bridge of the nose may help. Almost all nosebleeds can be controlled in this manner *if sufficient time is allowed for the bleeding to stop.*

Nosebleeds are more common in the winter, when both viruses and dry, heated air indoors are common. A cooler house and a vaporizer to return humidity to the air help many patients.

If nosebleeds are a recurrent problem, are becoming more frequent, and are not associated with a cold or other minor irritation, then a physician should be consulted on a nonurgent basis. The physician should not be seen immediately after the nosebleed since examination at that time may simply restart the nosebleed, resulting in wasted time and money.

What to Expect at the Doctor's Office

The patient will be seated, head back, and the nostrils compressed. This will be done even if the patient has been doing this at home, and it will usually work. Packing the nose or attempting to cauterize a bleeding point is less desirable. If the nosebleed cannot be stopped, the nose will be examined to see if a bleeding point can be identified. If a bleeding point is seen, coagulation by either electrical or chemical cauterization may be attempted. If this is not successful, then packing of the nose may be unavoidable. Such packing is uncomfortable, may lead to infection, and the patient must be carefully observed.

If a physician is seen because of recurrent nosebleeds, questions about events preceding the bleeds and a careful examination of the nose itself should be expected. Depending on the history and the physical examination, blood-clotting tests may be required.

Nosebleeds 20

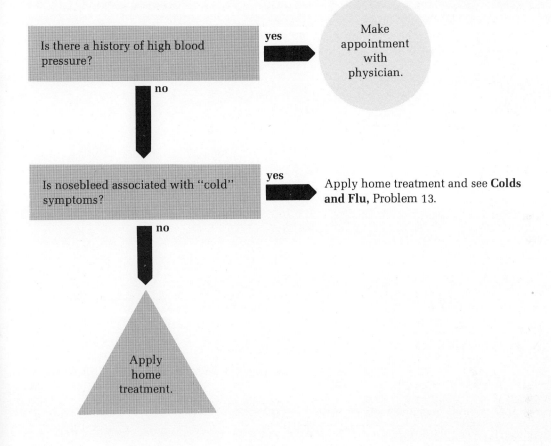

Is there a history of high blood pressure?

yes → Make appointment with physician.

no ↓

Is nosebleed associated with "cold" symptoms?

yes → Apply home treatment and see **Colds and Flu,** Problem 13.

no ↓

Apply home treatment.

F
Common Skin Problems

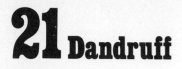

21 Dandruff

Dandruff is a common and simple problem. The common mistakes in diagnosis of these scaling lesions of the scalp are to call dandruff "psoriasis" or to miss another problem which is co-existing with the dandruff. In most cases, the distinction between psoriasis and dandruff is easily made. Psoriasis often stops at the hairline. Furthermore, the scales of psoriasis are on top of raised lesions called "plaques." The medical term for dandruff is "seborrhea." "Seborrheic dermatitis" is a long term for a skin disease which is equivalent to "dandruff" of the skin on other parts of the body.

Home Treatment

The heavily advertised anti-dandruff shampoos are helpful in mild or moderate cases of dandruff. For severe and more stubborn cases there are some less well-known over-the-counter shampoos which are effective. Selsun (available by prescription only) and Selsun Blue are brand names of shampoos which contain selenium sulfide; Selsun Blue is available over-the-counter and, while weaker, is just as good if you apply more of it more frequently. When using these shampoos, it is important that directions be followed carefully, as oiliness and yellowish discoloration of the hair may occur with their use. Sebulex, Sebucare, and Sebutone are another series of anti-dandruff preparations which also must be used strictly according to directions.

No matter what you do, the problem will probably come back, and you will have to repeat the treatment. If the problem gets worse despite home treatment over several weeks, see the doctor. You will not be going to the doctor for the usual case of dandruff.

What to Expect at the Doctor's Office

You will not be going to the doctor for dandruff. Very severe cases of seborrheic dermatitis can require more than shampoo, and a physician may prescribe topical cortisone or other treatment.

Are all of the following conditions present:

a) fine, white scales;

b) scaling confined to scalp and/or eyebrows;

c) only *mild* redness in involved areas?

 no → Suspect problem other than dandruff*

yes

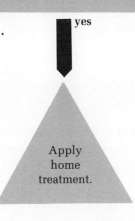

Apply home treatment.

* Rethink your condition and consult other Common Skin Problem charts in this section. All skin conditions are not listed, only the most common. If your condition has continued for several weeks with no relief, make an appointment with the doctor.

22 Poison Ivy & Poison Oak

Poison ivy and poison oak need little introduction. The itching skin lesions which follow contact with these and other plants of the Rhus family are the most common example of a larger category of skin problems known as "contact dermatitis." Contact dermatitis simply means that something has been applied to the skin which has caused the skin to react to it. An initial exposure is necessary to "sensitize" the patient; a subsequent exposure will result in an allergic reaction if the plant oil remains in contact with the skin for several hours. The resulting rash begins after 12 to 48 hours delay and persists for about two weeks. Contact may be indirect, from pets, contaminated clothing, or from smoke from burning Rhus plants. It *can* occur during any season.

Home Treatment

There are many approaches to the treatment of poison ivy. The best is to avoid the plants, which are hazardous even in the winter when they have dropped their leaves. Next best is to remove the plant oil from the skin as soon as possible. If the oil has been on the skin for less than six hours, thorough cleansing with strong soap, repeated three times, will usually prevent reaction.

Many physicians recommend cool compresses of Burrow's Solution (Domeboro, Bur-Veen, Bluboro) or Aveeno Bath (one cup to a tub full of water). The old standby, calamine lotion, is sometimes of help in early lesions, but may spread the plant oil which is causing the irritation to the skin in the first place. Be sure to cleanse the skin, as above, even if you are too late to prevent the rash entirely. Another useful method of obtaining symptomatic relief is the use of a hot bath or hot shower. Heat releases histamine, the substance in the cells of the skin which causes the intense itching. Therefore, a hot shower or bath will cause intense itching as the histamine is released. The heat is gradually increased to the maximum tolerable and continued until the itching has subsided. This process will deplete the cells of histamine and the patient will often obtain eight hours of relief from the itching. This method has the advantage of not requiring frequent applications of ointments to the lesions and is a good way to get some sleep at night. Poison ivy or oak will persist for the same length of time despite the medication. If secondary bacterial infection occurs, healing will be delayed; hence scratching is not helpful. Cut the nails to avoid damage to the skin through scratching.

If the lesions are too extensive to be easily treated, if home treatment is ineffective, and if the itching is so severe you just can't stand it, a visit to the physician may be necessary.

What to Expect at the Doctor's Office

After a history and physical examination, the physician may deal with poison ivy or oak in several ways, usually by prescribing a steroid cream to be applied four to six times a day to the lesions. This is often of moderate help. Another alternative is to give a steroid (such as prednisone) by mouth for short periods of time. A rather large dose is given the first day and the dose is then gradually reduced. Response to treatment may be disappointingly slow. The itching may be treated symptomatically either with an antihistamine (Benadryl, Vistaril) or a sedative. All medications which you may receive have their hazards. Prednisone or other steroids taken by mouth may cause emotional changes, ulcers, and other problems, and many physicians will not prescribe them for poison ivy or oak. The antihistamines may cause drowsiness and may make driving dangerous. You must judge whether your misery from the itching makes the significant risks of therapy worthwhile.

Poison Ivy
&
Poison Oak
22

Are all of the following conditions present:

a) itching;

b) redness, minor swelling, blisters, or oozing;

c) definite exposure to poison ivy, poison oak, or poison sumac?

no ⟶ Suspect problem other than poison ivy.*

yes

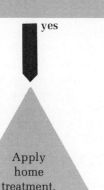

Apply home treatment.

* Rethink your condition and consult other Common Skin Problem charts in this section. All skin conditions are not listed, only the most common. If your condition has continued for several weeks with no relief, make an appointment with the doctor.

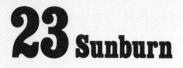

23 Sunburn

Sunburn is common, painful, and bears testimony to bad judgment. Very rarely, persons with sunburn have difficulty with vision; if so, they should visit their physician. Otherwise, do not see your doctor unless the pain is extraordinarily severe or unless blistering (not peeling) has occurred. Blistering indicates a second degree burn, and rarely follows sun exposure. The pain of sunburn is worst between 6 and 48 hours after sun exposure. Peeling of injured layers of skin occurs later—between three and 10 days after the burn.

Home Treatment

Cool compresses or cool baths with Aveeno (one cup to a tub full of water) may be useful. Ordinary baking soda (one-half cup to a tub) is nearly as effective. Lubricants such as Vaseline feel good to some patients, but retain heat and should not be used the first day. Avoid products which contain benzocaine. These may give temporary relief but can cause irritation of the skin and may actually prolong healing.

Sunburn is better prevented than treated. For protection, effective sunscreens are available. Protection is afforded by Block-out, Pabafilm, Pabonal, and Presun, among others.

What to Expect at the Doctor's Office

The physician will direct the history and physical examination toward determination of the extent of burn and the possibility of other heat-related injuries like sunstroke. If only first-degree burns are found, a prescription steroid lotion may be prescribed. This is not of particular benefit. The rare second-degree burns may be treated with antibiotics applied to the skin. Therapy may include pain relief with analgesics or sedation. There is no evidence that steroid lotions or antibiotic creams help at all in the usual case of sunburn; most physicians prescribe the same therapy available at home.

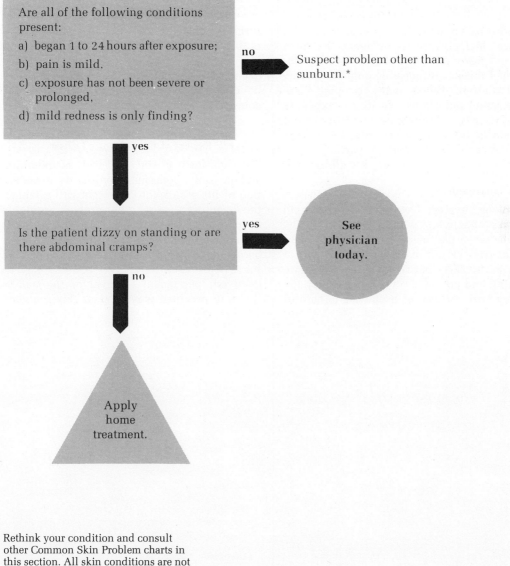

Are all of the following conditions present:

a) began 1 to 24 hours after exposure;

b) pain is mild,

c) exposure has not been severe or prolonged,

d) mild redness is only finding?

no → Suspect problem other than sunburn.*

yes

Is the patient dizzy on standing or are there abdominal cramps?

yes → See physician today.

no

Apply home treatment.

* Rethink your condition and consult other Common Skin Problem charts in this section. All skin conditions are not listed, only the most common. If your condition has continued for several weeks with no relief, make an appointment with the doctor.

24 Athlete's Foot

Athlete's foot is the most common of the fungal infections and is often persistent. When it involves toenails, it can be a difficult problem to treat. Friction and moisture are important in aggravating the problem. In fact, there is evidence that bacteria and moisture cause most of this problem; the fungus is responsible only for getting things started. When many people share locker room and shower facilities, exposure to this fungus is impossible to prevent; and infection is the rule, rather than the exception. But you don't have to participate in sports to contact this fungus; it's all around.

Home Treatment

Scrupulous hygiene, without resorting to drugs, is effective. *Twice a day:* wash the space between the toes with soap, water, and a cloth; dry the entire area carefully with a towel, particularly between the toes (despite the pain); and put on clean socks. Keeping the feet dry with the use of a powder is helpful in preventing reinfection. In difficult cases, over-the-counter drugs such as Desenex powder or cream may be used. The powder has the virtue of helping keep the toes dry. If these are not effective, a more expensive over-the-counter medication, Tinactin (tolnaftinate) is available in either cream, lotion, or powder form. Recently, the twice-daily application of a 30 percent aluminum chloride solution has been strongly recommended by some for its drying and antibacterial properties. You will have to ask your pharmacist to make up the solution, but it is inexpensive.

What to Expect at the Doctor's Office

Through history and physical examination, and possibly potassium hydroxide examination of the scales, the physician will establish the diagnosis. Several other problems, notably a condition called dyshydrosis, may mimic athlete's foot. An oral drug, griseofulvin, may occasionally be used but is not recommended for this problem. Rarely, the toenails may be involved; permanent removal of the nail is the only practical way to treat this problem.

Are all of the following conditions present:

a) redness, scaling between toes and on soles of feet only (may have cracks between toes and some small blisters);

b) age more than 10 years;

c) itching?

no Suspect problem other than athlete's foot*

yes

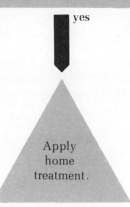

Apply home treatment.

* Rethink your condition and consult other Common Skin Problem charts in this section. All skin conditions are not listed, only the most common. If your condition has continued for several weeks with no relief, make an appointment with the doctor.

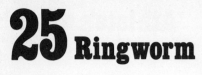

25 Ringworm

Ringworm is a fungus infection of the skin. Usually it is trivial but if it involves the scalp or nails, it can be slightly more serious. Ringworm of the scalp requires oral therapy with a prescription drug called griseofulvin. Other skin problems may be difficult to distinguish from ringworm. Fortunately, the home treatment of ringworm is reasonably safe, may even help other conditions, and will not cause harm if the diagnosis is not accurate. The principal features of ringworm are listed in the chart.

Home Treatment

Tinactin (tolnaftate) applied to the skin is an effective treatment for ringworm. It is available in cream, solution, and powder, and can be purchased over-the-counter. Either the cream or solution should be applied two or three times a day. Only a small amount is required for each application. Resolution of the problem may require several weeks of therapy but improvement should be noted within 7 days. Selsun Blue shampoo, applied as a cream several times a day, will frequently do the job as well and is much less expensive.

What to Expect at the Doctor's Office

The diagnosis of ringworm can be confirmed by taking a scraping of the scales, soaking them in a potassium hydroxide solution, and viewing them under the microscope. Since ringworm is a fungal disease, the fungal spores can be observed under the microscope. If lesions are extensive, involve the scalp, or are particularly resistant to local therapy, the physician may elect to treat with griseofulvin, taken by mouth. Ringworm of the scalp may be detected by a special light, called a Wood's lamp, which will cause affected hair to become fluorescent.

Are all of the following conditions present:

a) round, red, scaling lesions with more activity at periphery giving a ringlike appearance;

b) centers of lesions not filled in;

c) confined to chest, abdomen and back?

No → Suspect problem other than ringworm.*

Yes

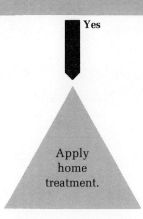

Apply home treatment.

---

* Rethink your condition and consult other Common Skin Problem charts in this section. All skin conditions are not listed, only the most common. If your condition has continued for several weeks with no relief, make an appointment with the doctor.

26 Jock Itch

We might wish for a less picturesque name for this condition, but "tinea cruris" is a term understood by relatively few. "Jock itch" is a fungus infection of the pubic region. It is aggravated by friction and moisture. It usually does not involve the scrotum or penis or spread beyond the groin area. For the most part, this is a male disease only.

Home Treatment

Tinactin may be used; the powder form is best. The problem should also be treated by removing the contributing factors, friction and moisture. This is done by using boxer type shorts rather than "Jockey" shorts, by applying a powder to dry the area after bathing, and by frequently changing soiled or sweaty underclothes. It may take up to two weeks to completely clear this problem, and it may recur. The powder and clean shorts treatment may be successful even without the medication.

What to Expect at the Doctor's Office

Occasionally a yeast infection will mimic "jock itch." By examination and history the physician will attempt to establish the diagnosis and additionally may make a scraping in order to identify a yeast. Medicines used for this problem are virtually always applied to the affected skin; oral drugs or injections are rarely used.

Are all of the following conditions present:

a) involves only groin and thighs;

b) redness, maceration or oozing, some peripheral scaling;

c) itching?

no ⟶ Suspect problem other than jock itch.*

yes

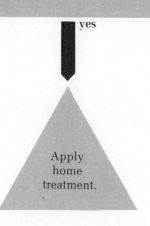

Apply home treatment.

* Rethink your condition and consult other Common Skin Problem charts in this section. All skin conditions are not listed, only the most common. If your condition has continued for several weeks with no relief, make an appointment with the doctor.

27 Patchy Loss of Skin Color

Tinea versicolor is a very shallow fungus infection which sits on the top layer of the skin, gives the appearance of loss of pigment, and is most apparent in the summer. The lesions may be fawn-colored. The clue to the diagnosis is the very fine scales that are present. There are no other symptoms—no itching, pain, or fever. Unfortunately, it always recurs.

Home Treatment

As with ringworm, this is a fungal disease and will respond to the application of Tinactin. The infection is so shallow and minor that it can also be removed by use of Selsun Blue shampoo applied daily to the affected skin, sudsed, and washed off. If you don't respond to this therapy within two weeks, make an appointment with your physician. Intermittent maintenance therapy, weekly or bi-weekly, is often required.

What to Expect at the Doctor's Office

The physician may elect to take a scraping of the fine scales, subject them to a potassium hydroxide solution, and view them under a microscope. The diagnosis is confirmed by the appearance of the fungal spores under the microscope. The diagnosis may also be made by determining that the affected skin glows under a special light called a Wood's lamp.

Therapy at the physician's office is the same as that available at home.

Are all of the following conditions present:

a) patient feels well.

b) lightly scaled, tan, pink, or white patches;

c) no redness or swelling;

d) confined to chest or back?

No Suspect problem other than fungus.*

Yes

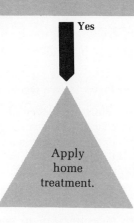

Apply
home
treatment.

* Rethink your condition and consult other Common Skin Problem charts in this section. All skin conditions are not listed, only the most common. If your condition has continued for several weeks with no relief, make an appointment with the doctor.

28 Acne

Acne is a superficial skin eruption which is caused by a combination of factors. As is well-known, it is a frequent problem in adolescence and in persons with oily skin. The increased skin oils of puberty accumulate below keratin plugs in the openings of the hair follicles and sweat glands. In this stagnant area below the plug, secretions accumulate and bacteria grow. The bacteria cause changes in the secretions which make them irritating to the surrounding skin. The result is usually a pimple, but sometimes may develop into a larger pocket of secretions, or cyst. Blackheads are formed when the plug is quite noticeable, and the irritation of the skin is minimal.

Home Treatment

The most effective preventive is cleanliness and hygiene. Soap and water, twice daily, will control the problem for most people. This does not mean that people with acne are less clean than those without. Rather, the rubbing and heat of the cloth help dislodge the keratin plug. The soap helps remove skin oil and decrease the number of bacteria living on the skin. Greases and creams on the skin may sometimes aggravate the condition. The various patent medicines available over-the-counter appear to help some people; they are disappointing in others. Diet is not an important factor in most cases, but if chocolates, nuts, or other foods tend to aggravate the problem, avoid them.

Several further steps may be taken at home if necessary. An abrasive soap, such as Pernox or Brasivol, may be used from one to three times daily to further reduce the oiliness of the skin and to remove the keratin plugs from the follicles.

A drying agent, such as Fostex, may be employed in the same manner but irritation may occur if it is used too often. Finally, natural sunlight or a sun lamp is effective if used conscientiously. Guidelines for the sunlamp are as follows:

- Use at a distance of 12 inches.
- Expose three sides of face in succession (left, center, right).
- Wear goggles or place damp cotton over eyes.
- Treat two or three times a week.
- Use a timer. Start at 30 seconds for each surface. Increase the exposure by 30 seconds at each exposure. Should a mild burn occur, discontinue for one week. Restart at one-half previous time.
- Do not read or sleep under a sunlamp.

Should these measures fail to control the problem, make an appointment with the physician.

What to Expect at the Doctor's Office

The physician will advise about hygiene and the use of medications. In resistant cases an antibiotic, tetracycline or erythromycin, may be prescribed to be taken by mouth.

All of the following conditions are present:

a) Pimples and/or blackheads only;

b) Confined only to face, chest and/or back;

c) No cysts or nodules?

no ▶ Suspect problem other than Acne.*

yes

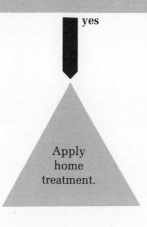

Apply home treatment.

* Rethink your condition and consult other Common Skin Problem charts in this section. All skin conditions are not listed, only the most common. If your condition has continued for several weeks with no relief, make an appointment with the doctor.

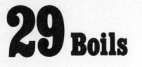

29 Boils

"Painful as a boil" is a familiar term and emphasizes the severe discomfort which can arise from this common skin problem. A boil is a localized infection due to the staphylococcus germ; usually a particularly savage strain of the germ is responsible. When this particular germ inhabits a person's skin, recurrent problems with boils may persist for months or years. Often several family members will be affected at about the same time. Boils may be single or multiple, and they may occur anywhere on the body. They range from the size of a pea to the size of a walnut or larger. The surrounding red, thickened and tender tissue increases the problem even further. The infection begins in the tissues beneath the skin, and develops into an abscess pocket filled with pus. Eventually, the pus pocket "points" toward the skin surface and finally ruptures and drains. Then it heals.

Special consideration should be given to boils on the face since they are more likely to lead to severe complicating infections.

Home Treatment

Boils are handled gently, because rough treatment can force the infection deeper inside the body. Warm, moist soaks are applied gently several times each day to speed the development of the pocket of pus and to soften the skin for the eventual rupture and drainage. Once drainage begins, the soaks will help keep the opening in the skin clear. The more drainage the better. Frequent thorough soaping of the entire skin helps prevent reinfection. Ignore all temptation to squeeze the boil.

What to Expect at the Doctor's Office

If there is fever or a facial boil, the doctor will usually prescribe an antibiotic. Otherwise, antibiotics may not be used; they are of limited help in abscess-like infections. If the boil feels like fluid is contained in a pocket, but has not yet drained, the physician may lance the boil. In this procedure, the skin is numbed with a local anesthetic and a small incision made to allow the pus to drain. After drainage the pain is reduced and healing is quite prompt. While "incision and drainage" is not a complicated procedure, it is tricky enough that you should not attempt it yourself.

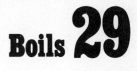
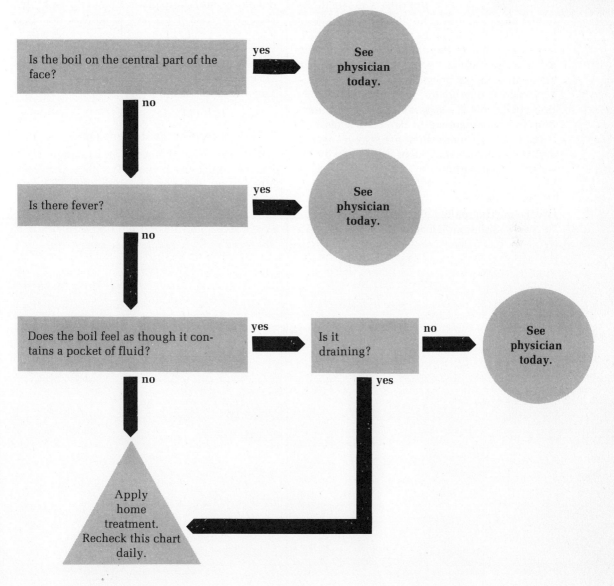

Is the boil on the central part of the face? — yes → **See physician today.**

no ↓

Is there fever? — yes → **See physician today.**

no ↓

Does the boil feel as though it contains a pocket of fluid? — yes → Is it draining? — no → **See physician today.**

no ↓   yes ↓

Apply home treatment. Recheck this chart daily.

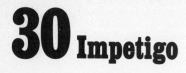

30 Impetigo

Most mothers are familiar with the characteristic, crusted-over sores of impetigo. For this one you need the doctor and antibiotics. Home treatment should be applied only in cases without fever, with sores only on the arms and legs, and with only a few lesions. Even then you must review the situation each 12 hours and check the chart again. Go to the doctor, if there is any question at all. This is a superficial bacterial infection which can spread to deeper tissues.

Impetigo is most common between ages 1 and 10. Do not assume the problem is impetigo outside this age group.

Home Treatment

Crusts may be soaked off with either water or Burrow's Solution (Domeboro, Bluboro). An antibiotic ointment (Bacitracin, Neosporin) may be applied. If lesions do not show *prompt* improvement or if they seem to be spreading, the patient should see the physician without delay. An antibiotic given by mouth or by injection is often necessary to control impetigo and prevent the kidney problems which sometimes follow such an infection. In infants, a staphylococcal impetigo may turn into a very severe infection of the entire skin surface.

What to Expect at the Doctor's Office

After examining the sores and taking an appropriate medical history, the physician usually will prescribe an oral antibiotic. The drug of choice is penicillin unless there is a history of sensitivity to penicillin, in which case erythromycin will usually be prescribed.

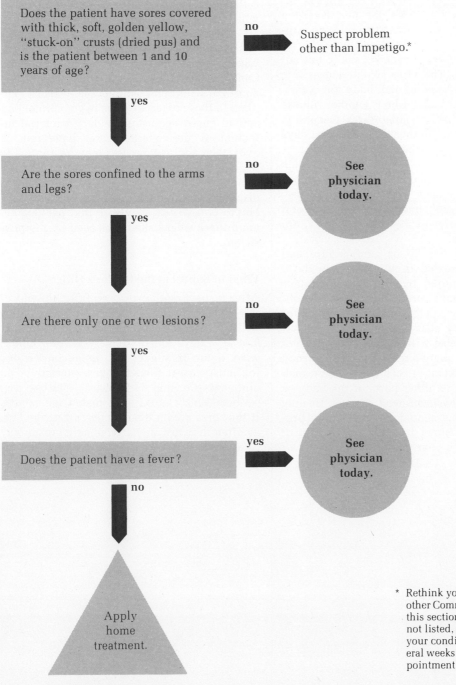

Does the patient have sores covered with thick, soft, golden yellow, "stuck-on" crusts (dried pus) and is the patient between 1 and 10 years of age?

no → Suspect problem other than Impetigo.*

yes ↓

Are the sores confined to the arms and legs?

no → **See physician today.**

yes ↓

Are there only one or two lesions?

no → **See physician today.**

yes ↓

Does the patient have a fever?

yes → **See physician today.**

no ↓

Apply home treatment.

* Rethink your condition and consult other Common Skin Problem charts in this section. All skin conditions are not listed, only the most common. If your condition has continued for several weeks with no relief, make an appointment with the doctor.

31 Cold Sores & Fever Blisters

Fever blisters are a familiar problem caused by a virus. They are usually found on the lips, although they can sometimes appear inside the mouth. Often the blisters have ruptured and only the remaining sore is seen. Fever is usually but not always present. The virus which causes this problem often lives in the body for years, causing trouble only when another illness causes a rise in body temperatures. Generally, fever blisters heal by themselves several days after the fever diminishes.

A canker sore often follows an injury such as accidently biting the inside of the lip or the tongue, or may appear without obvious cause. Both of these problems are self-limited and minor. More serious sores, paradoxically, are usually painless.

A cancer of the lip or gum is rare and need not be treated in the first few days. Syphilis transmitted by oral sexual contact may give a mouth sore. Both of these problems are usually painless. There are other conditions that may also give mouth ulcers, but also give problems with eyes, joints, or other organs. Rarely, allergic reactions to drugs may cause mouth ulcers; in such cases a skin rash will be present on other parts of the body as well, and the physician must be seen. Healing of mouth lesions should not be unduly prolonged; if any sores last more than two or three weeks, see your doctor.

Home Treatment

Since these sores heal by themselves the goal of therapy is relief of pain. A protective covering will often accomplish this. For sores inside the lip and on the gums a preparation called Orabase is available over-the-counter which may be applied to these sores and will give them protection. For cold sores and fever blisters on the outside of the lips, one of the phenol and camphor preparations (Blistex, Campho-Phenique) may provide relief. Neosporin or Bacitracin Ointment may also be applied to these external sores to give protection and to guard against secondary bacterial infection. If the external sores have crusted over, then cool compresses may be applied to remove the crusts. If one of these preparations appears to cause further irritation, then discontinue it. Mouth sores usually resolve in one to two weeks. Any sore that persists beyond three weeks should be seen by the physician.

What to Expect at the Doctor's Office

After inspecting the sore carefully, the physician may prescribe a special ointment which will help eliminate the virus if sores are in their first few days and extremely severe. Otherwise, home treatment will be recommended for most cases. Sometimes, a steroid in an ointment (Kenalog in Orabase) may be prescribed. This can be used inside the mouth. If the sores are on the outside part of the lips, as often they are, any steroid skin cream may be applied.

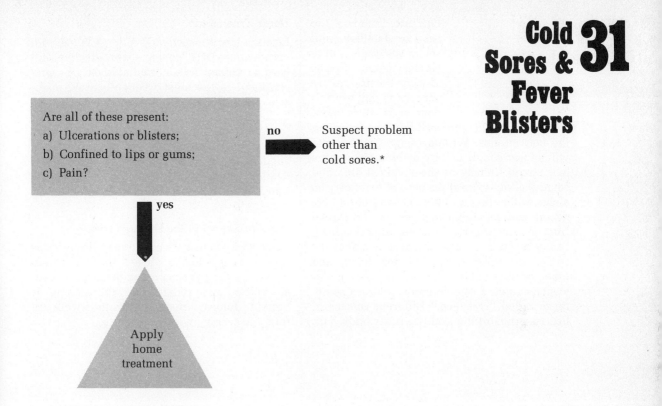

Are all of these present:
a) Ulcerations or blisters;
b) Confined to lips or gums;
c) Pain?

no → Suspect problem other than cold sores.*

yes

Apply home treatment

* Rethink your condition and consult other Common Skin Problem charts in this section. All skin conditions are not listed, only the most common. If your condition has continued for several weeks with no relief, make an appointment with the doctor.

32 Lice

Lice are found in the best of families, and social status is not a barrier to the disease. The lice themselves are very small and are seldom seen. It is more worthwhile looking to see if there are "nits" on the hair strands. Without magnification, nits will appear simply as tiny black lumps on the hair strand. Itching of the involved area and small shallow sores at the base of hairs may be a clue to the disease. Pubic lice are not a "venereal disease" although they may be spread from person to person during sexual contact. Unlike syphilis and gonorrhea, lice may be spread by toilet seats, infected linen, and other sources. Pubic lice, when seen under magnification, resemble crabs, and are sometimes called "crab lice." Different species of lice may inhabit the scalp or other body hair.

Home Treatment

Lice are small insects and may be killed with insecticides. DDT powders are effective, but hard to obtain. Kwell (available only by prescription) is the most frequently used medicine. Several over-the-counter medications, including A200 and Cuprex, are also effective for pubic lice. Instructions that come with these drugs must be followed carefully. Linen and clothing must be changed simultaneously. Sexual partners should be treated at the same time.

What to Expect at the Doctor's Office

Since Kwell is usually effective in lice infestations it is practically always the medication chosen by the physician. The diagnosis is usually clear and relief from the itching is prompt. Repeat treatments with Kwell are rarely necessary with proper use.

Are any of the following conditions present:

a) itching in scalp or pubic hair areas;

b) lice seen on skin or in clothing;

c) nits seen on hair shafts?

no → Suspect problem other than lice.*

yes

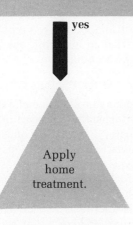

Apply home treatment.

* Rethink your condition and consult other Common Skin Problem charts in this section. All skin conditions are not listed, only the most common. If your condition has continued for several weeks with no relief, make an appointment with the doctor.

33 Skin Bumps & Lumps

Lumps and bumps on the skin cause a great deal of unnecessary concern. Usually, the worry is cancer. Only rarely is the problem serious, and treatment is seldom required. The lump may be above the skin, as in the case of warts and moles, within the skin as with boils and certain kinds of moles, or under the skin as in the case of small collections of fat called lipomas. If there is only one lump, and it is hot, red, swollen, and tender (inflamed), then it should be considered a boil until proven otherwise. (See Boils, Problem 29.) A dark mole which appears to be enlarging or changing color might be melanoma, a kind of skin cancer. However, few skin lesions which appear to be enlarging and changing color are cancer. All moles must start small and grow larger, and the removal of all moles is impossible as well as undesirable. Unfortunately, there is no easy way out of this dilemma because there is no certain way for a patient to identify a melanoma without the aid of a physician.

The more common skin cancers are found in persons of middle and older ages in sun-exposed areas of the skin. Usually skin cancer is not serious, but it may occasionally spread to other parts of the body. These cancers appear as nonhealing sores and should be shown to a physician. A more common recurrent problem in the same locations and in the same age range is "actinic keratosis," which is an irregular, brownish, raised, scaly lesion. Actinic keratosis is not cancerous but, on occasion, it will become malignant. Thus some physicians advocate observing these lesions for change or bleeding, while others recommend removal. We usually watch and wait.

Home Treatment

The rational approach to a skin lump is to observe it to see if it changes size or color, bleeds, or gets inflamed. Otherwise, don't worry so much. In the absence of these characteristics the only reason to have lesions removed is for cosmetic purposes. Warts can be removed with commercially available over-the-counter preparations if used consistently and carefully (Compound W, Vergo). On your next routine visit to a doctor, ask about any skin lumps which bother you.

What to Expect at the Doctor's Office

The physician may be able to make the diagnosis simply by inspecting the wart or lump and obtaining a history. If a major question of diagnosis remains, a "punch" biopsy may be taken. This type of biopsy removes a portion of the bump for examination under the microscope. Alternatively, the entire lump may be removed. This approach may be desirable for cosmetic reasons or because of a potentially serious skin problem.

Warts may be removed by freezing with liquid nitrogen or by using an electric needle. In contrast to other skin problems, they are seldom removed surgically since they are caused by viruses and cutting them out may leave the virus to cause a recurrence of the wart later. Even under the best of circumstances, recurrence of warts is a familiar problem and repeated treatments may be necessary.

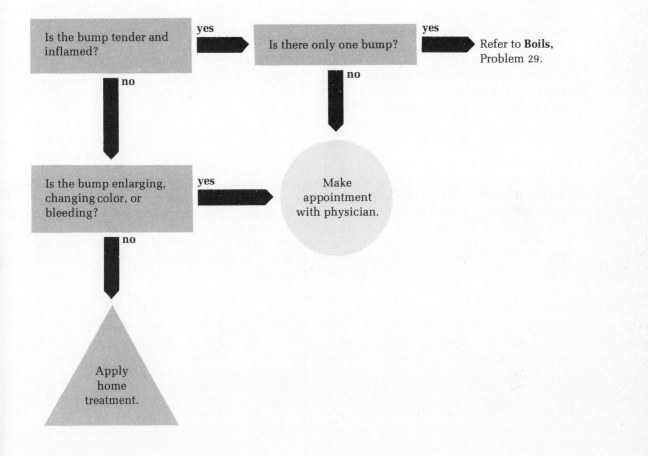

Is the bump tender and inflamed? — **yes** → Is there only one bump? — **yes** → Refer to **Boils**, Problem 29.

no ↓

no ↓

Is the bump enlarging, changing color, or bleeding? — **yes** → Make appointment with physician.

no ↓

Apply home treatment.

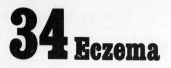

34 Eczema

Eczema is one of the most common skin conditions as well as one of the most frustrating to treat. Because of its persistence, most patients with eczema will see a physician at some time during the illness. The main purpose of this chart is to reinforce understanding of the problem as well as the principles of its therapy. The characteristics of eczema are given in the chart. Because of a tendency to run in families, it will often be recognized by an older family member when it makes its appearance in a younger member.

Home Treatment

The key point to remember about eczema is that it is a result of having skin which is very easily damaged. Eczema is simply a sign of skin which will not take much abuse. A person with eczema must come to realize that soap, chemicals, and other drying agents are harmful to the skin rather than helpful. Bathing must be kept to a minimum and exposure to agents which irritate the eczema must be avoided. Also avoid rough clothing such as wool. Avoid overheating when possible. Use rubber gloves or other types of protection to avoid contact with agents toxic to the skin. When you must use soap stay with a very gentle soap such as Lowilla. Cetaphil Lotion may be used as a cleansing agent.

What to Expect at the Doctor's Office

By history and examination of the lesions, the physician can determine whether the problem is eczema. The mainstay of treatment is steroid cream and lotions. While these are effective, they are not curative and eczema is characterized by repeated occurrences. During periods of severe problems, the use of a steroid cream or lotion will often be necessary. If the sores do not appear typical of eczema or if the disease runs an unusual course, it may be necessary to perform a biopsy to be certain of the diagnosis. Secondary infection is not rare and antibiotics are sometimes required.

Are all of the following conditions present:

a) oozing, moist, red lesions;

b) localized to elbows, wrists, knees, or around eyes;

c) age below 20;

d) personal or family history of asthma, eczema, hayfever, or hives?

 no

Suspect problem other than Eczema.*

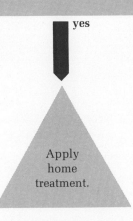 **yes**

Apply home treatment.

* Rethink your condition and consult other Common Skin Problem charts in this section. All skin conditions are not listed, only the most common. If your condition has continued for several weeks with no relief, make an appointment with the doctor.

G
Childhood Diseases

SHOTS, IMMUNIZATIONS, AND KEEPING UP-TO-DATE

The term, "usual childhood diseases," is unfortunate in several respects, but does convey some of the characteristics of these problems. Grandmother has traditionally diagnosed and prescribed for these illnesses, and probably has done as well as or better than most physicians. Today, the increasing belief that every illness should be seen by a physician has resulted in these diseases becoming a prime source of unnecessary visits to the physician. There are several good reasons *not* to go to the doctor:

- These viral illnesses have no cure. The doctor can help only with complications.

- These illnesses are contagious. You may expose other patients.

- You neglect grandmother. Let her take a look. (Just make sure she has read this book first if she is out of practice.)

Preventive medicine is the best medicine. Immunization protects against several of the diseases in this section. In addition, immunization is effective against several other diseases which are a good deal more sinister: diphtheria, pertussis (whooping cough), tetanus (lockjaw), polio, and smallpox. The standard sequence of immunizations is given at the back of the book; space is provided to record the dates that the shots were given. Note that routine immunization against smallpox is no longer recommended (although this is presently controversial). If you have not had the basic immunizations listed, contact your physician as to the appropriate action. In general, everyone should be immunized against diphtheria, tetanus, and polio.

35 Chicken Pox

How to recognize the chicken pox.

Before the rash: Usually there are no symptoms before the rash, but occasionally there is fatigue and some fever in the 24 hours before the rash is noted.

The rash: The typical rash goes through the following stages.

a. First it appears as flat red splotches;

b. They become raised and may resemble small pimples;

c. They develop into small blisters, called vesicles, which are very fragile. They may look like drops of water on a red base. The tops are easily scratched off.

d. As the vesicles break, the sores become "pustular" and form a crust. (The crust is made of dried serum, not true pus.) This stage may be reached within several hours of the first appearance of the rash. The crust falls away between the ninth and thirteenth day. Itching is often severe in the pustular stage.

e. The vesicles tend to appear in crops with two to four crops appearing within two to six days. All stages may be present in the same area. They usually appear first on the scalp and in the mouth, then spread to the rest of the body. They are most numerous over shoulders, chest, and back. They are seldom found on the palms of the hands or the soles of the feet. There may be only a few sores, or there may be hundreds.

Fever: After most of the sores have formed crusts, the fever usually subsides.

Chicken pox spreads very easily—over 90 percent of brothers and sisters catch it! It may be transmitted from 24 hours before the appearance of the rash up to about 6 days after. It is spread by droplets from the mouth or throat or by direct contact with contaminated articles of clothing. It is not spread by dry scabs. The incubation period is from 14 to 17 days. Chicken pox leads to life-long immunity to recurrence with rare exceptions. However, the same virus which causes chicken pox also causes shingles and the individual with a history of chicken pox may develop shingles later in life.

Most of the time, chicken pox should be treated at home. Rarely, there may be complications which require a physician. The specific questions on the chart deal with two severe complications which may require more than home treatment, encephalitis (viral infection of the brain) and severe bacterial infection of the lesions. Encephalitis is rare.

Home Treatment

The major problem in dealing with chicken pox is control of the intense itching and reduction of the fever. Warm baths containing baking soda (½ cup to a tubful of water) frequently help. The use of antihistamines (Benadryl) or other sedatives is sometimes necessary and may require contact with your physician; check by phone before exposing other children in a doctor's office.

Cut the fingernails or use gloves to prevent skin damage from intensive scratching. When lesions occur in the mouth, gargling with salt water (½ teaspoon salt to an eight-ounce glass) may help comfort and will cleanse the lesions. Hands should be washed three times a day and all of the skin should be kept gently but scrupulously clean in order to prevent a complicating bacterial infection. Minor bacterial infection will respond to soap and time; if it becomes severe and results in return of fever, then see the physician. Scratching and infection can result in permanent scars.

What to Expect at the Doctor's Office

Do not be surprised if the physician is willing and even anxious to treat the case "over the phone." Chicken pox is a contagious disease and other children should be protected if possible. If it is necessary to bring the patient to the doctor's office, then attempts should be made to keep him or her separate from the other children. In healthy children chicken pox has few lasting ill effects, but in children with other serious illnesses it can be a devastating or even fatal disease. A visit to the physician's office should not be recommended unless a complication seems possible.

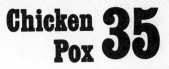
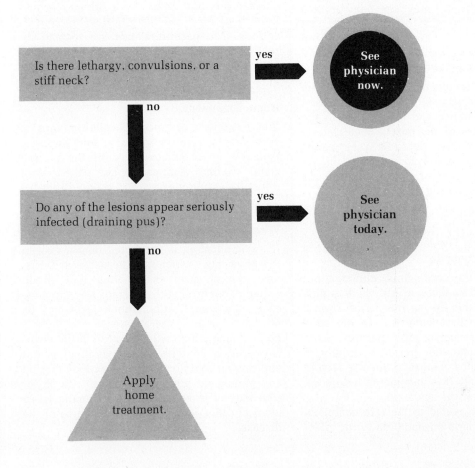

Is there lethargy, convulsions, or a stiff neck?

yes → See physician now.

no

Do any of the lesions appear seriously infected (draining pus)?

yes → See physician today.

no

Apply home treatment.

36 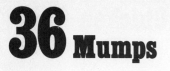Mumps

How to recognize the mumps:

Before the salivary glands swell: There may be one or two days of low fever and malaise. Chewing and swallowing may produce pain behind the ear. Sour substances make the pain worse.

Salivary gland involvement: Swelling of the parotid glands causes the characteristic "mumps" appearance and lasts seven to ten days. Tenderness of the mouth usually lasts only for one to three days. Salivary glands under the jaw and tongue may also be involved. The openings of the glands into the mouth may become red and puffy.

Fever: May be as high as 104°F, or there may be none.

Other symptoms: Headache, fatigue, and loss of appetite are common.

Mumps is quite contagious, although not as easily spread as measles and chicken pox. It is communicable during the period from 2 days before the first symptoms to the complete disappearance of the parotid gland swelling. The incubation period is usually 16 to 18 days. Mumps is most frequently seen in winter and spring. It is uncommon before the age of 3 and after the age of 40.

The chart is directed to the rare complications which include encephalitis (viral infection of the brain), pancreatitis (viral infection of the pancreas), kidney disease, deafness, and involvement of one or both testicles. Complications are more frequent than in chicken pox but are unusual. Adults, particularly men, are more likely to develop complications. The parotid glands are located directly in front of the ear. Swelling of these glands gives the familiar "chipmunk" appearance to the face.

Home Treatment

The treatment of uncomplicated mumps is very simple: Aspirin for fever and for pain. Isolation is recommended until the parotid gland swelling disappears. The patient with difficulty eating may require a liquid diet for a few days.

What to Expect at the Doctor's Office

If a complication is suspected then a visit to the physician's office may be necessary. History and physical examination will be directed at confirming the diagnosis or the presence of a complication. Blood tests may be needed. Mumps is a viral disease, and there is no medicine which will directly kill the virus. However, even with extensive involvement and several complications, the outlook is good and permanent problems are rare. The physician may offer additional symptomatic treatment but this does not alter the course of the disease.

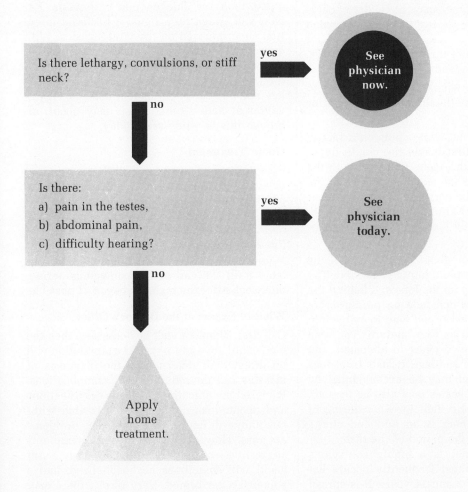

Is there lethargy, convulsions, or stiff neck?

yes → See physician now.

no ↓

Is there:
a) pain in the testes,
b) abdominal pain,
c) difficulty hearing?

yes → See physician today.

no ↓

Apply home treatment.

37 Measles (Rubeola)

How to recognize the measles:

Three to five days before the rash: There may be a dry, "barking" cough, inflamed eyes (watery, but not draining pus), a sore throat, a nasal discharge, and swollen neck glands.

Fever: The fever, which ranges from 101° to 104°, also occurs in the three to five days prior to the rash.

Koplik's spots: Fine, white spots on a faintly red base appear first inside the mouth opposite the molar teeth. Again, these occur in the three or four days immediately preceding the rash. There may be only one or two spots, or they may cover the entire inside of the mouth. These spots usually fade as the skin rash appears.

Rash: Appearing on about the fifth day of the illness, the rash is pink, blotchy, and flat. The spots first show up on the face and behind the ears. The spots, which fade on pressure, become somewhat darker and tend to merge into larger red patches as they mature. The rash spreads from head to chest to abdomen, and finally to the arms and legs. It lasts from four to seven days and may be accompanied by mild itching. Fine scales may also be present. There may be some light brown coloring of the skin. Often there is an odd and strong body odor during the period of the rash.

Measles (rubeola) is a highly contagious viral disease. It most frequently occurs between the ages of 2 and 14 years. It is spread from person to person by droplets from the mouth or throat and by direct contact with articles freshly soiled by nose and throat secretions. It may be spread during the period from three to six days before the appearance of the rash to one week after the onset of the rash. The incubation period is eight to twelve days with the majority of cases occurring approximately ten days after exposure.

Specific questions in the chart are addressed to complications; these are more frequent than for chicken pox or mumps. Ear pain and cough may signal a bacterial infection superimposed on the viral measles. With appropriate therapy complications are usually minor. However, measles encephalitis (viral infection of the brain) is a very serious problem and can cause permanent damage. Aggravation of active tuberculosis may occur, although this is rarely seen today.

Home Treatment

Symptomatic measures are all that is required or available. Aspirin should be used for temperature greater than 102°F, and a vaporizer should be used for cough. Saline gargles may be of help. If the eyes are involved, then saline sponges and dim light may make a child more comfortable. The child should be isolated until the end of the contagious period, one week after the rash has begun, if possible.

What to Expect at the Doctor's Office

Call first. Should a visit be necessary, then the medical history and physical examination will be directed at determining the diagnosis of measles and the nature of any complications. Bacterial complications, such as ear infections and pneumonia, can usually be treated without undue difficulty and persistent problems are rare. However, the child with symptoms suggestive of encephalitis (lethargy, stiff neck) will sometimes be hospitalized, and a spinal tap performed. Very rarely, there may be a problem with blood clotting so that abnormal bleeding occurs. Usually, this is first apparent as dark purple splotches in the skin. Measles is a viral disease, and there is no drug which specifically kills the virus. However, professional supportive therapy is important with severe complications.

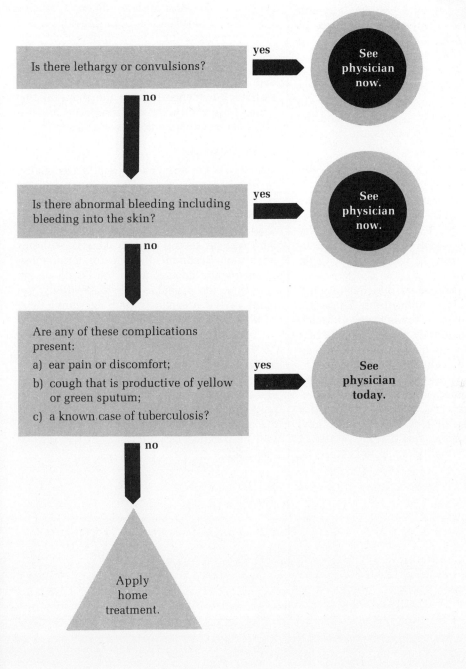

Is there lethargy or convulsions?

yes → See physician now.

no ↓

Is there abnormal bleeding including bleeding into the skin?

yes → See physician now.

no ↓

Are any of these complications present:
a) ear pain or discomfort;
b) cough that is productive of yellow or green sputum;
c) a known case of tuberculosis?

yes → See physician today.

no ↓

Apply home treatment.

38 German Measles (Rubella, Three-day Measles)

How to recognize the German measles:

Before the rash: There may be a few days of mild fatigue. Lymph nodes at the back of the neck may be enlarged and tender.

Rash: The rash first appears on the face as flat or slightly raised red spots. It quickly spreads to the trunk and the extremities and the discrete spots tend to merge into large patches.

Fever: The fever rarely goes above 101°F and usually lasts less than two days.

German measles (rubella) is a mild virus infection which is not as contagious as measles or chicken pox. It is usually spread by droplets from the mouth or throat. The incubation period is from 12 to 21 days with an average of 16 days.

The specific questions on the chart are addressed to possible complications. These are essentially the same as for measles although they occur less frequently and are usually less serious. In addition, patients with rubella may have swelling and aching in several joints.

The main concern with German measles is not the usual disease in a child but infection in an unborn child. If three-day measles occurs during the first month of pregnancy, there is a 50 percent chance that the fetus will develop an abnormality such as cataracts, congenital heart disease, deafness, or mental deficiency. By the third month of pregnancy this risk is decreased to less than 10 percent and it continues to decrease throughout the pregnancy. Because of this problem, a vaccine for German measles has been developed, and is recommended for children between the ages of one year and puberty. There has been some controversy concerning this vaccine; however, the controversy involves questions of statistical evidence beyond the scope of this manual. Currently, the great majority of pediatricians recommend the rubella vaccine.

Home Treatment

Usually no therapy is required. Occasionally, fever will require the use of aspirin. Isolation is usually not imposed. Avoid any exposure to women who could possibly be pregnant. If a question of such exposure arises, the pregnant woman should discuss the risk with her physician. Recommendations for termination of pregnancy depend upon the length of the exposure, the probable risk to the fetus, the point in the pregnancy, and the convictions of the prospective parents.

What to Expect at the Doctor's Office

Visits to the physician's office are seldom required for uncomplicated German measles. Questions about possible infection of pregnant women are more easily and economically discussed over the telephone. Complications will be handled essentially as in the case of measles.

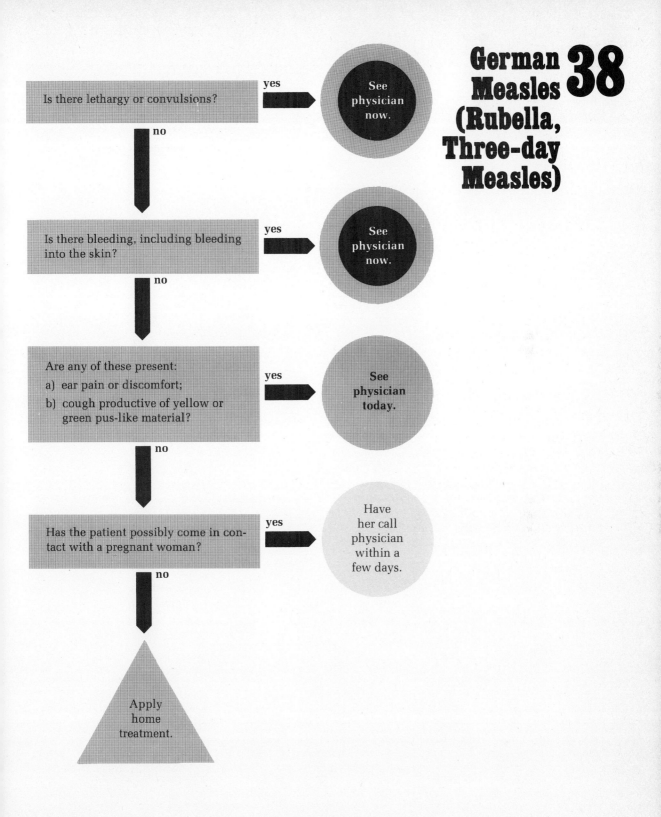

Is there lethargy or convulsions?

yes → See physician now.

no ↓

Is there bleeding, including bleeding into the skin?

yes → See physician now.

no ↓

Are any of these present:
a) ear pain or discomfort;
b) cough productive of yellow or green pus-like material?

yes → See physician today.

no ↓

Has the patient possibly come in contact with a pregnant woman?

yes → Have her call physician within a few days.

no ↓

Apply home treatment.

German 38 Measles (Rubella, Three-day Measles)

169

H
Arthritis, Back Pain, and Other Aches and Pains

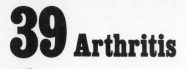

39 Arthritis

Most "arthritis" is not arthritis at all! Misunderstanding comes from a different use of the term by doctors and by patients. The "arth" part of the word means "joint"—not muscle, tendon, ligament, or bone. The "itis" means "inflamed." Thus, true arthritis affects the joints, and the joints are red, warm, swollen, and painful to move. Pains in the muscles or ligaments are discussed in Problem 41.

There are over one hundred types of arthritis and you cannot be sure which type you have. The four most common types are "osteoarthritis," "rheumatoid arthritis," "gout," and "ankylosing spondylitis." Osteoarthritis is usually not serious, occurs in later life, and frequently causes knobby swelling at the most distant joints of the fingers. Rheumatoid arthritis usually starts in middle life and may cause you to feel sick and stiff all over, in addition to the joint problems. Gout occurs mostly in men, with sudden, severe attacks of pain and swelling in one joint at a time—frequently the big toe, the ankle, or the knee. Ankylosing spondylitis affects the back and joints of the lower back and may be suspected if your back is sore for a long time, particularly stiff in the morning, and you are unable to touch your toes.

Only rarely does a patient with arthritis need to be seen by a physician immediately. Home treatment and patience will usually resolve the problem shortly. The relative emergencies are (1) infection, (2) nerve damage, (3) fractures near a joint, and (4) gout. In the first three, serious damage may result if the joint is neglected; in the fourth the pain is so intense that immediate help is needed.

Contrary to popular belief, most kinds of arthritis can be treated. If arthritis persists more than six weeks, see a physician.

The complications of arthritis and treatment for arthritis occur very slowly and are more easily prevented than corrected. Arthritis results in more lost workdays and sickness than any other disease category—it must be managed correctly and with care.

Home Treatment

Aspirin is more powerful than prescription drugs for most patients with arthritis but only when used in high doses continued for a long period. Aspirin can reduce the swelling in the joints as well as the pain. For adult patients the usual dose is three to four tablets (15–20 grains) every four hours, for a total of 12 to 16 tablets daily. If this dose causes ringing in the ears, dizziness, or affects hearing, it is too high and should be reduced. Upset stomach usually can be avoided by taking the aspirin after meals, after an antacid (Maalox or Gelusil) or by using coated aspirin tablets (Ecotrin, A.S.A. Enseals). While aspirin has fewer side effects than most drugs, a physician should monitor treatment with these doses if it is maintained for several weeks or longer. Note that aspirin substitutes (acetaminophen) do *not* have the anti-inflammatory property of aspirin. (See Chapter 7)

Resting an inflamed joint can speed healing. Heat may help. Usually, a painful joint should be worked through its entire range of motion twice daily to prevent later stiffness or contracture.

What to Expect at the Doctor's Office

The physician will examine the joints, take several blood tests, and, often, x-ray the involved joint areas. If a joint contains fluid, the fluid may also be removed and tested. A cortisone-like drug may be injected (not more than three times) into a painful joint. Beware of the long-term oral use of such drugs—their side effects may be worse than the arthritis. If such drugs as prednisone are to be continued for more than a few weeks, we recommend that a consultant concur in their use. The good physician will invariably use aspirin or one of the "nonsteroidal anti-inflammatory agents" (such as indomethacin) before resorting to cortisone or its derivatives.

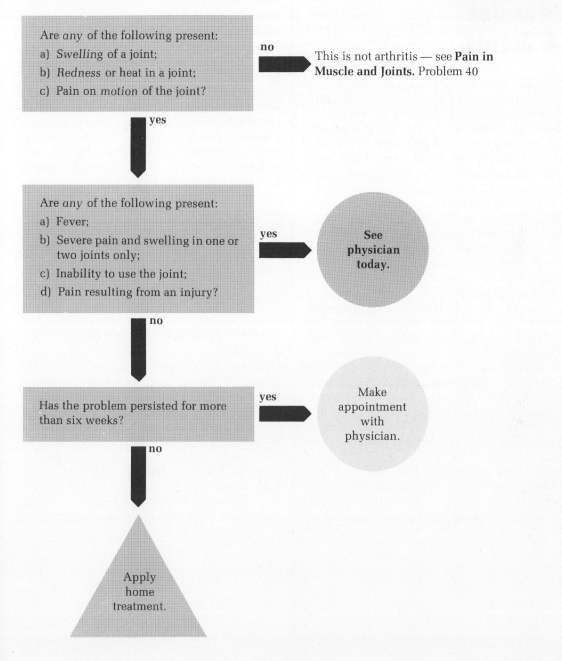

Are *any* of the following present:
a) *Swelling* of a joint;
b) *Redness* or heat in a joint;
c) Pain on *motion* of the joint?

no → This is not arthritis — see **Pain in Muscle and Joints.** Problem 40

yes

Are *any* of the following present:
a) Fever;
b) Severe pain and swelling in one or two joints only;
c) Inability to use the joint;
d) Pain resulting from an injury?

yes → **See physician today.**

no

Has the problem persisted for more than six weeks?

yes → Make appointment with physician.

no

Apply home treatment.

40 Pain in the Muscles & Joints

Here are two new medical terms: "arthralgia" means pain (without inflammation) in the joints, and "myalgia" means pain in the muscles. These pains are *not* "arthritis" but can be very bothersome. Usually they are not serious, and will go away. They can be caused by tension, virus infections, unusual exertion, automobile or other accidents, or can be without obvious cause. Only seldom do they indicate a serious disease. Rarely, thyroid disease, cancer, polymyositis (inflammation of the muscles), or, in older patients, a newly-known disease termed "polymyalgia rheumatica" may cause arthralgias. If fever, weight loss, or severe fatigue are not present, give home treatment a trial of several weeks or even months before seeing a physician. If pain is pronounced at the upper neck and base of the skull, the problem is almost certainly minor.

Doctors often do not agree on diagnostic terms in this area, and two doctors may give different names to your problem. Some terms frequently used are: "fibrositis," "nonarticular rheumatism," "chronic muscle-contraction syndrome," "psychogenic rheumatism," and "psycho-physiological musculo-skeletal pain." These all mean about the same. Medical treatment is often not very helpful. Tranquilizers, muscle relaxants, and pain relievers may be prescribed, but the side effects are often more spectacular than the relief provided. The doctor is frequently unsure whether the problem is physical or emotional in origin. These problems are "diseases of civilization" and are rarely seen in underdeveloped societies.

Home Treatment

Both rest and exercise are important. Try to relax and gently stretch the involved areas. Warm baths, massage, and stretching exercises should be used as frequently as possible. Sponge-soled shoes may help if you work on hard floors. Better light or a better chair may help if you work at a desk. Regular exercise (slowly increased from very gentle to more vigorous) may help restore the proper muscle tone. We recommend walking, bicycling, and swimming. Aspirin, two tablets (10 grains) four times daily may help—higher doses usually are of no additional benefit. If aspirin is poorly tolerated, acetaminophen (Tylenol) may be substituted in the same dosage. A change in life style or a move to a different location is frequently followed by improvement. If the problem goes away on vacation, you can be relatively certain that everyday stress accounts for the problem.

What to Expect at the Doctor's Office

A physical examination. Often, some blood tests. Rarely, x-rays. Advice similar to that above. In general, pain relievers containing narcotics or codeine are not useful. Oral corticosteroids such as prednisone should almost never be used unless a specific diagnosis can be made. If a particular spot in the body is causing the pain, a corticosteroid injection into that area may help greatly; such injections should not be repeated if they do not help and should be repeated only two or three times even if they do give prolonged relief.

Are any of the following present:

a) *Swelling* of a joint;

b) *Redness* or *heat* in a joint;

c) Pain on *motion* of the joint?

yes See **Arthritis,** Problem 39.

no

Are any of the following present?

a) Fever not associated with "flu" symptoms.

b) Weight loss of 10 or more pounds.

c) Fatigue or pain lasting more than three weeks?

yes → Make appointment with physician.

no

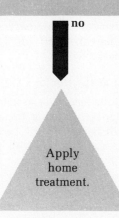 Apply home treatment.

41 Low-back Pain

Few problems can frustrate patient and physician alike as much as "low-back pain." The pain is slow to resolve and apt to recur. The frustration then becomes a part of the problem and may also require treatment.

Low-back pain usually involves spasm of the large supportive muscles alongside the spine. Any injury to the spine or back may produce such spasms; pain (often severe) and stiffness result. The onset of pain may be immediate or may occur some hours after the exertion or injury. Often the cause is not clear.

Most muscular problems in the back are linked to some exertion or lifting and must heal naturally; give them time. Back pain that results from a severe blow or fall may require immediate attention. As a practical matter, if back pain is caused by an injury received at work a physician is required by the Workman's Compensation laws.

The most common location of pain due to muscular strain is in the low back. Although many other pains have a muscular origin, pain that extends beyond the low-back area suggests a need for concern. Pain which seems to travel down one leg is very different than pain confined to the low back. Leg pain suggests pressure on the nerves as they leave the spinal cord and requires the help of a physician. If backache occurs with other symptoms (such as difficult periods), refer to the appropriate chart for that symptom.

Home Treatment

The low-back-pain syndrome is a vicious cycle in which injury causes muscle spasm, the spasm induces pain, and the pain results in additional muscle spasm. Therapy helps disrupt this cycle. Muscle spasm is intended to immobilize an injured part; sometimes it increases the problem.

Resting the muscles is of primary importance. When the pain first appears, rest, flat on your back, for at least 24 hours. Follow the period of complete bed rest by a gradual increase in activity, carefully avoiding reinjury. Severe muscle-spasm pain usually lasts for 48 to 72 hours and is followed by days or weeks of less severe pain. Strenuous activity during the next six weeks can bring the problem back and delay complete recovery. After healing, an exercise program will help prevent reinjury. No drug will hasten healing; they only reduce symptoms.

The patient should sleep, pillowless, on a very firm mattress, with a bedboard under the mattress, on a waterbed, or he or she may even be most comfortable on the floor. A folded towel beneath the low back may increase comfort.

Heat applied to the affected area will provide some relief. Two to three aspirin every three hours should be continued as long as there is significant pain. To avoid upset stomach, take the medication with milk or food or use buffered aspirin (Ascriptin, Bufferin, etc.).

There is little sound medical information on this subject. The advice given here is standard. If there is no nerve damage, hospitalization and the physician have little to offer. We have seen severe low-back syndromes where the patient ignored all advice and seemed to do just as well.

What to Expect at the Doctor's Office

Expect the physician or his assistant to ask questions similar to those on the chart. The examination will center on the back, the abdomen, and the extremities, with special attention to testing the nerve function of the legs. If the injury is the result of a fall or a blow to the back, x-rays are indicated; otherwise usually not. X-rays do not show injury to muscles, only to bones. If the history and the physical examination are consistent with lower back strain, the physician's advice will be similar to that described above. A muscle relaxant may be prescribed, but this is not definitely superior to aspirin. If the history and physical examination indicate damage to the nerves leaving the spinal cord, a special x-ray may be necessary. Only if nerve damage is present or the condition fails to heal for a prolonged period should hospitalization, traction, or surgery be required.

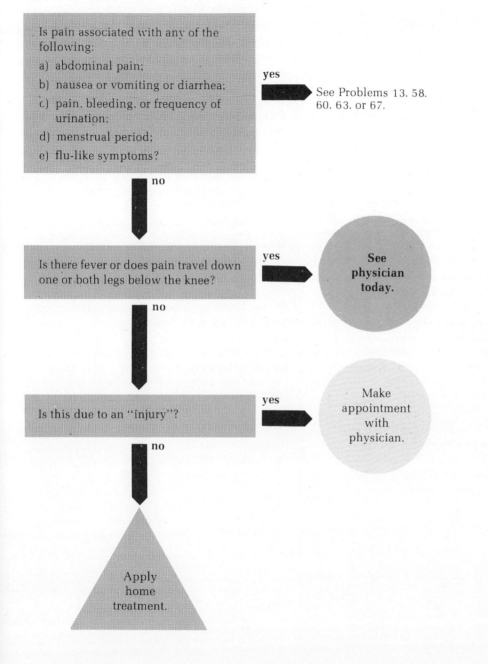

Is pain associated with any of the following:

a) abdominal pain;

b) nausea or vomiting or diarrhea;

c) pain, bleeding, or frequency of urination;

d) menstrual period;

e) flu-like symptoms?

yes → See Problems 13, 58, 60, 63, or 67.

no

Is there fever or does pain travel down one or both legs below the knee?

yes → See physician today.

no

Is this due to an "injury"?

yes → Make appointment with physician.

no

Apply home treatment.

42 Neck Pain

Most neck pain is due to strain and spasm of the neck muscles. The common "crick in the neck" on arising is one example of neck muscle strain. This type of neck pain can be adequately treated at home. Neck pains which require the attention of the physician include those due to meningitis or a pinched nerve.

With fever and headache there is a possibility of meningitis. More commonly, neck pain is part of a "flu" syndrome with fever, muscular aches, and a headache. When generalized aching throughout the muscles is present, a visit to a physician will seldom be useful. Meningitis may cause intense spasm of the neck muscles and a very stiff neck. When stiff neck is due to one of the more common causes of muscle spasm, the patient usually can touch the chin to the chest, even if with difficulty. If in doubt, it is better to see the physician for an ordinary muscle spasm than to attempt to treat meningitis at home.

Arthritis in the neck can result in a pinched nerve. When this is the cause of neck pain, the pain may extend down the arm, or there may be numbness or tingling sensations in the arm or hand. This pain is only on one side, and neck stiffness is not prominent.

Home Treatment

Neck pain in the morning means poor sleeping habits. Sleep on a firm surface and discontinue use of a pillow. A firm mattress is best. If this is not possible, then a bed-board will make the present mattress firmer. Warmth may be of benefit in relieving spasms and pain. Heat may be applied with hot showers, hot compresses, or a heating pad. Heat may be used as often as practical; don't burn the skin. Aspirin or acetaminophen (Tylenol, Tempra), two tablets every four hours, will help relieve pain and inflammation. Neck pain, like back pain, is slow to improve and may take several weeks to resolve. If an ordinary bath towel is folded lengthwise to a long four-inch wide strip, wrapped around the neck at bedtime and secured with tape or a safety pin, relief obtained overnight is often striking.

What to Expect at the Doctor's Office

If meningitis is suspected, the physician will perform a spinal tap as well as several blood tests. If a pinched nerve is likely, x-rays of the neck will be done. A muscle relaxant may be prescribed and perhaps a more powerful pain reliever. Valium is a frequently prescribed muscle relaxant. Prescription drugs are not necessarily better than aspirin; usually you are just as well off with home therapy if no infection or nerve damage is present.

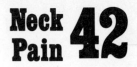

Neck Pain 42

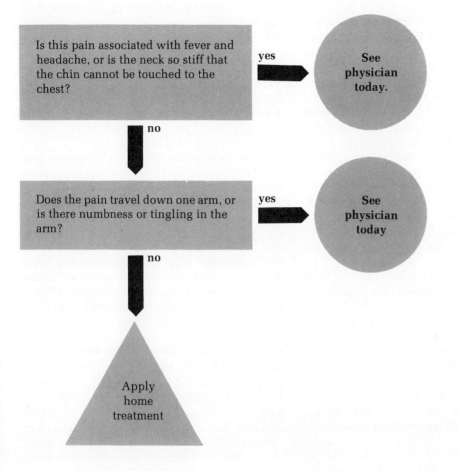

Is this pain associated with fever and headache, or is the neck so stiff that the chin cannot be touched to the chest?

yes → See physician today.

no

Does the pain travel down one arm, or is there numbness or tingling in the arm?

yes → See physician today

no

Apply home treatment

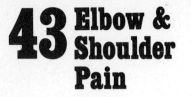

43 Elbow & Shoulder Pain

Pain located around the elbow or shoulder is common and almost never poses a serious threat to life. Nonetheless, it can persist for a long time and cause discomfort and disability. Most of the time the pain comes from the "soft tissues" near the joint and not from the bones or the joint itself. These soft tissues include the ligaments, the tendons, and the "bursae"—small pockets of special tissue which separate and lubricate the cartilage and bones that form the joint. Medical terms for these conditions include "bursitis," "tendonitis," "calcific tendonitis," and the self-descriptive "tennis elbow" and "frozen shoulder." If the hand and shoulder, but not the elbow, are involved, a rather unusual problem, the "shoulder-hand syndrome," may be present and the physician should be consulted.

Therapy for these conditions is not very advanced. Usually, a physician recommends home treatment, and reserves injection and surgery for only the very worst and long-lasting problems. Prescription medications are *not* predictably effective. The physician should be seen if the condition is very severe, if a fracture or dislocation is suspected, or if home treatment fails to relieve the problem. Unfortunately, you may be just as unhappy with the results of your physician's remedies.

Home Treatment

Irritation and inflammation of these soft tissues subsides with rest and time and becomes worse with active use of the involved part. Usually, about six weeks is required for the tissues to fully heal. If the part is too rigidly immobilized, two tissues may stick together (adhesion) during healing, resulting in permanent loss of a portion of the normal range of motion. Thus, treatment is designed not only to rest the part but to exercise it enough to prevent adhesions.

The activity which caused the problem (such as tennis-playing or heavy lifting) should be discontinued. An arm sling may be used to rest both shoulder or elbow. Gentle heat may speed healing. Carefully work the shoulder or elbow through its range of motion twice daily to preserve mobility. This is best done immediately after application of heat or a warm bath or shower. Aspirin or acetaminophen (Tylenol), two tablets (10 grains) every four hours, may be taken as needed.

Some authorities in sports medicine feel that problems related specifically to tennis or golf swings are treated more appropriately with lessons from the local pro than with pills from the local doctor. Poor sports technique results in most of these strains. This approach is well worth considering. The pro should be less expensive than the doctor and at least you can expect some help with your game.

As noted in the chart, the physician should be seen if the condition persists beyond six weeks.

What to Expect at the Doctor's Office

Examination of the affected area. General suggestions similar to those above. If pressure at a particular place reproduces most of your pain, injection of a corticosteroid medication into that area sometimes gives relief. Even if they work, two or three injections is plenty; many prominent athletes, particularly baseball pitchers, have had joints destroyed by a combination of continuing the irritating activity and using steroid injections to keep the inflammation down. Oral cortisone-like drugs or narcotic pain relievers are generally *not* indicated. Common sense and good medical practice both require that local problems be treated with local therapies if possible.

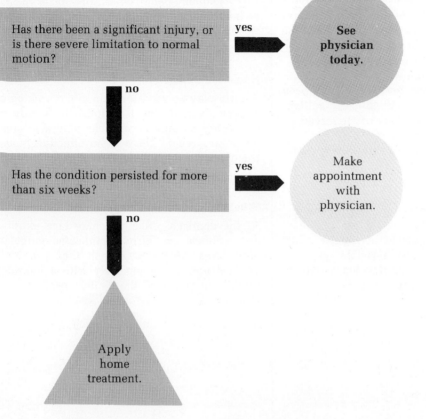

Has there been a significant injury, or is there severe limitation to normal motion?

yes → **See physician today.**

no

Has the condition persisted for more than six weeks?

yes → Make appointment with physician.

no

Apply home treatment.

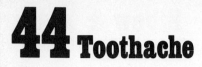

44 Toothache

Physicians often consider toothaches a frustrating and irritating problem. The physician cannot deal with the cause of the problem and can only suppress the pain with analgesics. Those who have the necessary skills, dentists, sometimes are difficult to find at night or on weekends.

Toothache often follows long-standing neglect of dental hygiene, and could have been prevented by a more enlightened patient. Minor, intermittent pain has often served as a warning of what was to come.

In general, you can avoid this unhappy situation by

- following a program of regular dental check-ups and oral hygiene, and

- preparing for the time when you may need a dentist outside of regular office hours. Discuss this possible problem with your dentist and develop a reliable method for obtaining dental help.

Write the appropriate phone numbers both on the chart and in the back of this book. Establish this after-hours procedure *before* you need it. Relying on the local emergency room may be a painful mistake.

Occasionally pain from ear or sinuses seems to involve the upper teeth. Treatment of the ear or sinus congestion will relieve this pain.

Home Treatment

Aspirin may be used for pain while seeking a dentist. Even if this is helpful, it is only a temporary measure. Ice packs may also give temporary relief. There is no effective home treatment for this problem.

What to Expect at the Dentist's Office

At the dentist's office you may face extractions, fillings, or fairly complicated surgical procedures. Makes you wish that you had brushed your teeth regularly with a fluoride toothpaste and used the dental floss!

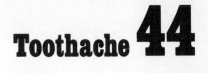
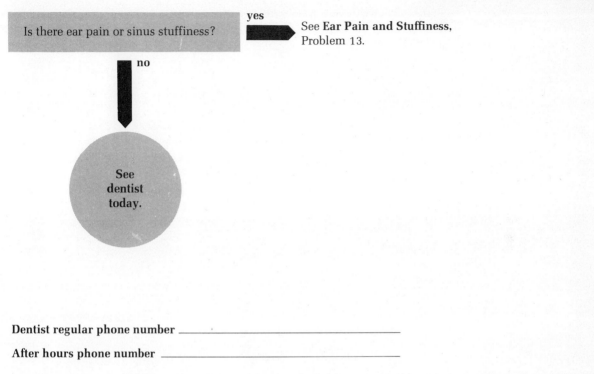

Is there ear pain or sinus stuffiness?

yes → See **Ear Pain and Stuffiness,** Problem 13.

no

See dentist today.

Dentist regular phone number _____

After hours phone number _____

I
Nervousness and Nerve Problems

45 Stress, Tension & Anxiety

Stress is a normal part of our lives. It is not necessarily good or bad. It is not a disease. Reactions to stress can vary enormously, and some of these reactions are undesirable. The most frequent undesirable reaction is anxiety. The degree of anxiety is much more a function of the individual than of the degree of stress. A person who reacts with excessive anxiety to everyday stress has a personal rather than a medical problem. The person who does not recognize anxiety as the problem will have difficulty in solving the problem.

Some common symptoms of anxiety are insomnia and lack of attention at work; these symptoms can lead to a vicious cycle which aggravates the situation. But the symptoms are effects, not causes, and the person who focuses on the insomnia or the lack of concentration as the cause of the problem is far away from a solution.

Most communities have several resources which can help with problems of anxiety. Ministers, social workers, friends, neighbors, and family may each play a beneficial role. The physician is an additional resource, but not necessarily the first or the best place to seek help for these problems.

Grief is an appropriate reaction to certain situations, such as death of a loved one or loss of a job. In such cases, time is the healer although significant help may be gained from the various family and community resources. Working through grief is an important part of getting over a loss. If the reaction persists several months, seek outside help.

The limitations of drugs such as tranquilizers or alcohol in this situation must be understood. While they may provide short-term symptomatic relief, they are brain depressants which do not enhance mental processes or solve problems. They are a crutch. In this instance, the long-term use of a crutch insures that the person using it will become a cripple. The underlying problem must be confronted.

Home Treatment

An honest attempt to identify the cause of the anxiety is a necessary first step in resolving the problem. When physical symptoms are due to job pressures, marital woes, wayward children, or dominating parents, the situation must be accurately identified, admitted, and confronted. When anxiety or depression is reactive, the cause is often obvious, and simply talking about it with friends or counselors will help. In other instances, identifying the source of the anxiety will be difficult, painful, time-consuming, and may eventually require the help of a professional counsellor or psychiatrist. Unfortunately, no scientific studies have been able to show better results with any particular type of therapy. So pay your money and take your choice.

Additionally, sometimes these symptoms are simply an overdose of one of the minor poisons of everyday life—caffeine. Watch out for coffee if you drink more than four cups a day, and remember that No-Doz, APC's, and a variety of cold and headache remedies contain caffeine.

What to Expect at the Doctor's Office

The family physician will attempt to identify the problem and to determine if the help of a psychiatrist or psychiatric social worker is required. Personal questions may be asked, and frank, honest answers must be given. Try to report the underlying problems and to avoid emphasis on the effects such as insomnia, muscle aches, headache, or inability to concentrate.

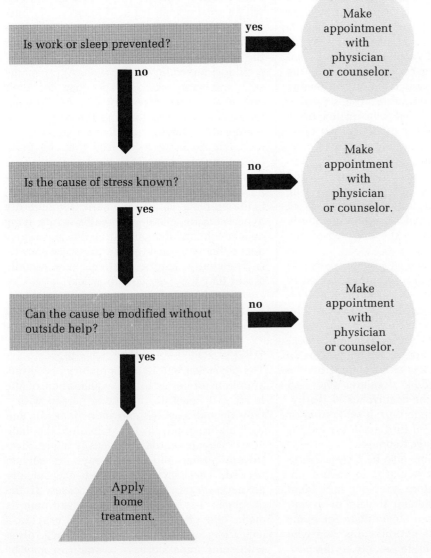

Is work or sleep prevented?

yes → Make appointment with physician or counselor.

no

Is the cause of stress known?

no → Make appointment with physician or counselor.

yes

Can the cause be modified without outside help?

no → Make appointment with physician or counselor.

yes

Apply home treatment.

46 The Hyperventilation Syndrome

Anxiety, especially unrecognized anxiety, can lead to physical symptoms. The hyperventilation syndrome is such a problem. In this syndrome a nervous or anxious person begins to be concerned by his or her breathing and rapidly develops a feeling of inability to get enough air into the lungs. This is often associated with a feeling of chest pain or constriction. The sensation of being out-of-breath leads to further over-breathing and a lowering of the carbon dioxide level in the blood; carbon dioxide is present in exhaled air. The lower level of carbon dioxide gives symptoms of numbness and tingling of the hands and of dizziness. The numbness and tingling may extend to the feet and also may be noted around the mouth. Occasionally, spasms of the muscles of the hands may occur.

This syndrome is almost always a disease of young adults. While it is more common in women it is also frequently seen in men. Usually, this syndrome occurs in persons who recognize themselves as nervous and tense. It often occurs when such persons are subjected to additional stress, to alcohol, or to situations where there is an advantage for the patient to have a sudden dramatic illness. A classical example is the occurrence of the hyperventilation syndrome during separation or divorce proceedings, so that a call for help is sent out to the estranged spouse.

Hyperventilation may also be a response to severe pain, and particularly to severe abdominal pain. Therefore an older individual or a person with abdominal pain or severe pain of any type is not a candidate for home treatment. When in doubt, take a person who is hyperventilating due to anxiety to the physician's office rather than discount a potentially serious problem because it is associated with hyperventilation.

Home Treatment

The symptoms of the hyperventilation syndrome are due to the loss of carbon dioxide into the atmosphere as a result of the over-breathing. If the patient breathes into a paper bag, so that the carbon dioxide is taken back into the lungs rather than being lost into the atmosphere, the symptoms will be alleviated. This usually requires five to fifteen minutes with a small paper bag held loosely over both the nose and the mouth. This is not always as easy as it sounds, since a major feature of the hyperventilation syndrome is panic and a feeling of impending suffocation. Approaching such a person with a paper bag for their mouth and nose may prove to be difficult, unless one can first reassure the patient.

Repeated attacks may occur. Once the patient has honestly recognized that the problem is anxiety rather than an organic disease, the attacks will stop because the panic component will not occur. Convincing the patient is the problem. Having the patient voluntarily hyperventilate (50 deep breaths while lying on a couch) and demonstrating that this reproduces the symptoms of the previous episode is frequently helpful. Patients are usually afraid that they are having a heart attack or are on the verge of a nervous breakdown. Neither is true, and when fear is dissipated hyperventilation usually ceases.

What to Expect at the Doctor's Office

The physician will obtain a history and direct attention primarily to the examination of the heart and lungs. In the young person with a typical syndrome, without abdominal pain and with a normal physical examination, the diagnosis of hyperventilation is easily made. Electrocardiograms and chest x-rays are seldom needed. These procedures may occasionally be necessary in less clear-cut cases. If the diagnosis of hyperventilation syndrome is made, the physician will usually provide a paper bag and the instructions above, often with some impatience. A tranquilizer may be administered; we prefer merely to reassure the patient. It is seldom possible to deal effectively with the cause of the anxiety during the hyperventilation episode. The patient should not assume that the underlying problem is solved simply because the hyperventilation has been controlled.

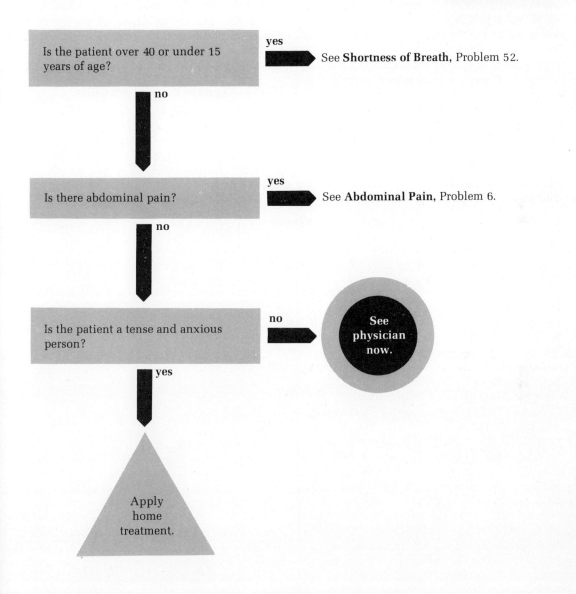

Is the patient over 40 or under 15 years of age?

yes → See **Shortness of Breath**, Problem 52.

no

Is there abdominal pain?

yes → See **Abdominal Pain**, Problem 6.

no

Is the patient a tense and anxious person?

no → See physician now.

yes

Apply home treatment.

47 Lump in the Throat

The feeling of a "lump in the throat" is the best known of all anxiety symptoms. There may even be some difficulty swallowing, although eating is possible if an effort is made. The sensation is intermittent, and is made worse by tension and anxiety. The difficulty in swallowing is worst when the patient concentrates on swallowing and on the sensations within the throat. As an experiment, try to swallow rapidly several times without any food or liquid, and concentrate on the resulting sensation. You will then understand this symptom.

Several serious diseases can cause difficulty in swallowing. In these cases, difficulty in swallowing begins slowly, is noticed first with solid foods and then with liquids, results in loss of weight, and is more likely to be found in those over 40. Lump-in-the-throat, like hyperventilation syndrome, is likely to be found in young adults, most frequently women.

Home Treatment

The central problem is not the symptom, but rather the underlying cause of the anxiety state. See the discussion of Anxiety, Problem 45. Recognition that the symptom is minor is crucial to its disappearance.

What to Expect at the Doctor's Office

After taking a medical history and examining the throat and chest, a physician occasionally may feel that x-rays of the esophagus are necessary. If an abnormality of the esophagus is found, further studies of the esophagus may be performed. The treatment given will probably be reassurance.

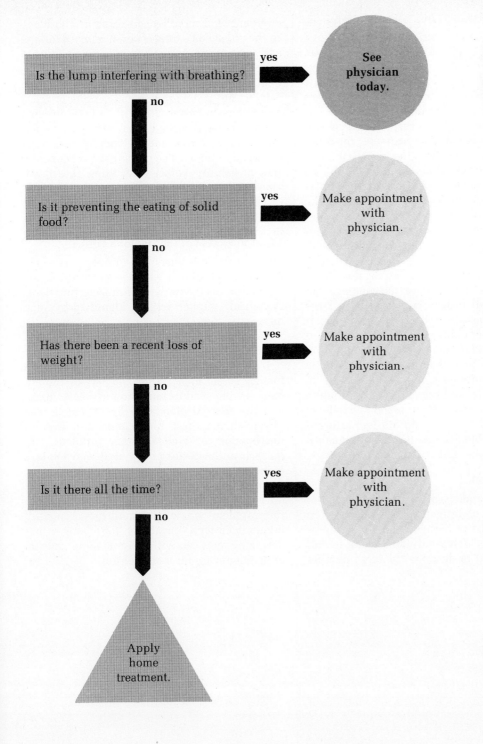

Is the lump interfering with breathing?

yes → **See physician today.**

no

Is it preventing the eating of solid food?

yes → Make appointment with physician.

no

Has there been a recent loss of weight?

yes → Make appointment with physician.

no

Is it there all the time?

yes → Make appointment with physician.

no

Apply home treatment.

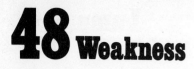

48 Weakness

Weakness and fatigue are often considered similar terms, but in medicine they have distinct and separate meanings. Weakness refers to lack of strength. Fatigue is tiredness, lack of energy, or lethargy. Although the chart uses the word "weakness" to indicate either complaint, the medical distinction between the two problems is preserved. Weakness is particularly important when it is confined to one area of the body, as in a "stroke."

Lack of energy, on the other hand, is associated typically with a virus infection or with a feeling of anxiety, depression, or tension. Weakness in one area is often due to a problem in the muscular or nervous system, whereas general fatigue is caused by a large variety of illnesses, especially those which create anxiety or depression.

Hypoglycemia means "low blood sugar" and many patients fear that this problem is the cause of their tiredness. A few individuals do in fact feel shaky and tremulous several hours after a meal because their blood sugar level drops at that point. They do *not* feel fatigued however. Low blood sugar throughout the day can cause fatigue, but it is very, very rare.

Home Treatment

There is time and need for careful reflection on the causes of fatigue. The most common situation has been termed "the tired housewife syndrome." This out-dated slang is still sometimes used to describe the large number of young and middle-aged women who come to the physician's office complaining of fatigue and requesting tests for anemia or thyroid problems. Many adult women are mildly iron-deficient, and thyroid problems may cause fatigue, but it is very unusual for one of these conditions to be the cause of fatigue. In most cases fatigue is more closely related to boredom, unhappiness, and disappointment than to organic factors. The patient should consider this possibility before consulting the physician with the problem of fatigue.

Vitamins are only very rarely helpful, but in moderation they do not hurt.

What to Expect at the Doctor's Office

If the problem is weakness of only part of the body, the physician will concentrate the examination on the nerve and muscle functions. A typical "stroke" will be identified by such an examination, whereas more uncommon ailments may require further testing and special procedures.

If the problem is fatigue, then the medical history is the most important part of the encounter. Physical examination of heart, lungs, and the thyroid gland can be expected. The physician may test for anemia and thyroid dysfunction, as well as other problems. Inquiry into the patient's life style and feelings is important. There are no direct cures for the most common fatigue syndromes. "Pep pills" *do not work,* and the rebound usually makes the problem worse. Tranquilizers generally intensify fatigue. Vacations, job changes, undertaking new activities, or making marital adjustments are far more helpful.

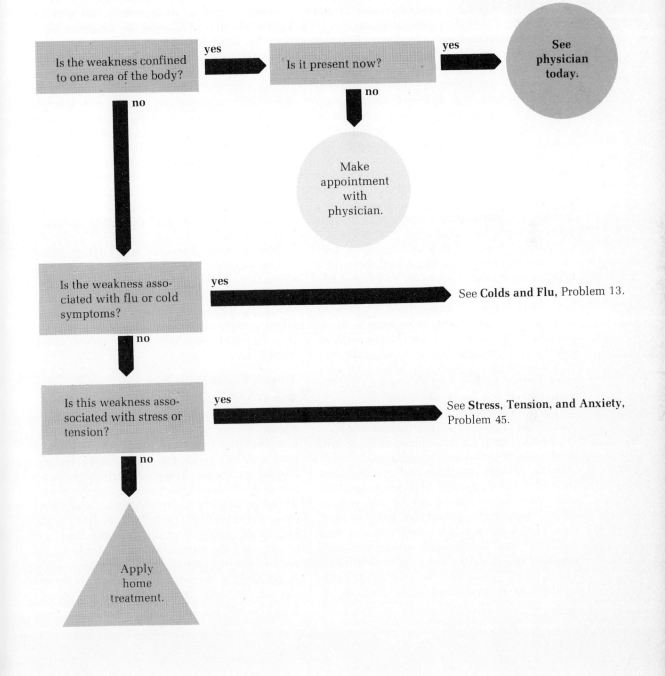

Is the weakness confined to one area of the body?

yes → Is it present now? **yes** → See physician today.

no ↓

Is it present now? **no** ↓ Make appointment with physician.

Is the weakness associated with flu or cold symptoms?

yes → See **Colds and Flu**, Problem 13.

no ↓

Is this weakness associated with stress or tension?

yes → See **Stress, Tension, and Anxiety**, Problem 45.

no ↓

Apply home treatment.

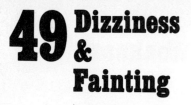

49 Dizziness & Fainting

Three different problems are frequently introduced by the complaint of dizziness or fainting: loss of consciousness, vertigo, and lightheadedness.

True unconsciousness includes a period in which the patient has no control over his body and of which there is no recollection. Therefore, if consciousness is lost while standing, the patient will fall and may sustain injury in doing so. The common symptom of "blackout" in which the patient finds it difficult to see and needs to sit or lie down but can still hear is not true loss of consciousness. Such "blackouts" may be related to changes in posture or to emotional experiences. True loss of consciousness may be caused by a number of conditions and needs to be investigated promptly by a physician.

"Vertigo" is caused by a problem in the balance mechanism of the inner ear. Since this balance mechanism also helps to control eye movements, there is not only loss of balance but also a feeling that the room is spinning around. Walls and floors may seem to lurch in crazy motions. Most vertigo has no definite cause and is thought due to a viral infection of the inner ear. A physician should be seen since further studies may be needed, and the vertigo itself may be totally disabling.

"Lightheadedness" is by far the most common of these problems. It is that woozy feeling which is such a common part of flu or cold syndromes. If such a feeling is associated with other flu or cold symptoms, refer to Problem 13. Lightheadedness which is not associated with other symptoms is usually not serious either. Many such patients are tense or anxious. Others have a low blood pressure and regularly feel lightheaded when suddenly standing up. This does not require treatment, and is called "postural hypotension." If lightheadedness is associated with the use of drugs, then the physician should be contacted to determine if the drug should be discontinued. Alcohol is a frequent cause.

Home Treatment

"Postural hypotension" is probably the most common cause of momentary blackout or lightheadedness. This problem becomes more frequent with increasing age. Typically, the patient notices a transient loss of vision or a lightheaded feeling when going suddenly from a reclining or sitting position to upright posture. The symptoms are caused by a momentary lack of blood flow to the brain. Most persons will experience this phenomenon at one time or another. The therapy is to avoid sudden changes in posture. Unless postural hypotension becomes suddenly worse, it alone is not sufficient reason for a separate visit to the physician. It may be reported on the next routine visit unless it is extremely frequent and troublesome.

Persons who experience a persistent lightheaded feeling without other symptoms should be reassured that this is not an indication of brain tumor or other hidden disease. This type of lightheadedness often disappears when anxiety is resolved. Not infrequently it is a problem with which the patient must learn to live.

What to Expect at the Doctor's Office

The physician will obtain a history with emphasis on making the distinctions outlined above. If loss of consciousness is the problem, then the heart and lungs will be examined and the nerve function will be tested. Special testing for irregular heartbeat or sudden drop of blood pressure may be necessary. If vertigo is the problem, then the head, ear, eyes, and throat will be examined, along with neurologic testing. Sometimes further tests of hearing or balance may be required. Medicine used to control vertigo can cause drowsiness. A search for predisposing factors, such as anxiety, will be made. Often a period of watchful waiting will be advised.

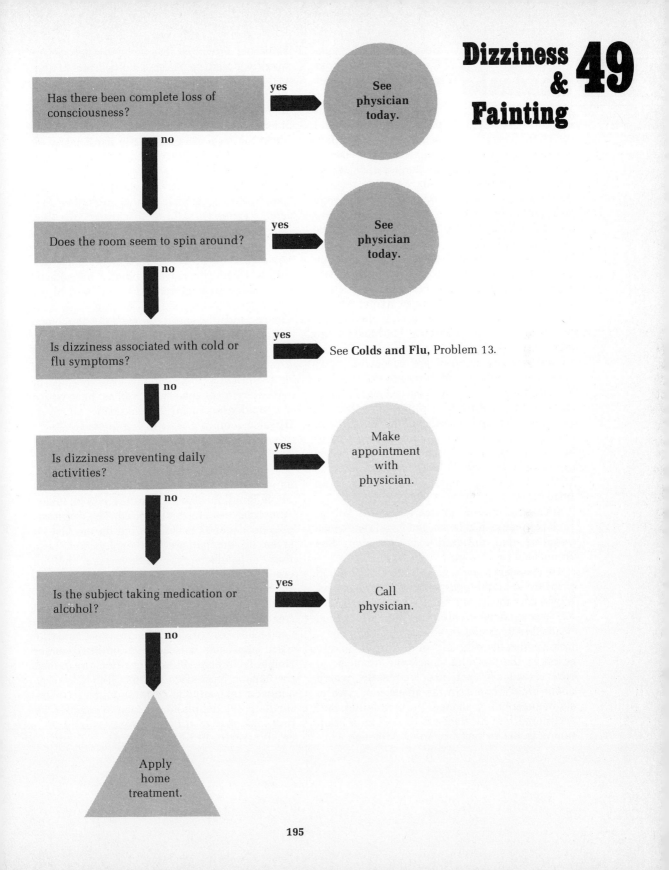

Has there been complete loss of consciousness? — yes → **See physician today.**

no ↓

Does the room seem to spin around? — yes → **See physician today.**

no ↓

Is dizziness associated with cold or flu symptoms? — yes → See **Colds and Flu,** Problem 13.

no ↓

Is dizziness preventing daily activities? — yes → Make appointment with physician.

no ↓

Is the subject taking medication or alcohol? — yes → Call physician.

no ↓

Apply home treatment.

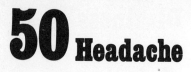

50 Headache

Headache is the most frequent single complaint of modern times. Most commonly, the causes are tension and muscle spasms in the neck, scalp, and jaw. For this reason, massaging or otherwise relaxing neck muscles can help relieve headaches. Most tension headaches will respond to the simple measures outlined below. Headache *without any other associated symptoms* is almost always caused by tension. Fever and a neck so stiff that the chin cannot be touched to the chest suggest the possibility of meningitis rather than an ordinary tension headache. But meningitis is rare even with these symptoms. Flu is much more likely. Muscle aches and pains are seldom seen in meningitis.

Most so-called "migraine" headaches are really severe tension headaches. True migraine headaches often are associated with nausea or vomiting and often are preceded by visual phenomena such as seeing "stars." They are caused by constriction and then relaxation of blood vessels in the head. True migraine headaches occur *only* on one side of the head during any particular attack. Drugs which constrict the blood vessels, such as Cafergot, will help migraine but not tension headaches.

Increased internal pressure due to head injury can cause headache and may also cause vomiting and difficulties with vision. See Problem 8.

Headache is not a reliable indicator of blood pressure. A high-blood-pressure headache usually occurs in the morning; tension headaches are more common later in the day. When headaches increase in severity or frequency, involve the back or top of the head, or are worst in the morning, check the blood pressure. Headache patients frequently worry about brain tumors. In the absence of paralysis or personality change, the possibility that an intermittent headache is caused by a brain tumor is exceedingly remote. Although constant and slowly increasing headaches are frequently noted in patients with brain tumors, it is usually some other symptom which leads the physician to institute an investigation for tumor. Headache patients should not be routinely investigated for possible brain tumor, since the tests are both costly and hazardous.

Home Treatment

Aspirin is the superdrug. Use it or another pain-killing drug such as acetaminophen (Tylenol, Tempra). All of the usual over-the-counter drugs are quite effective in relieving headache. Aspirin may be taken with milk or some food in order to prevent stomach irritation. Headache may frequently be relieved by massage or heat applied to the back of the upper neck or by simply resting with eyes closed and the head supported. Persistent headaches which do not respond to such measures should be brought to the attention of a physician. Headaches which are associated with difficulty in using the arms or legs or with slurring of speech, as well as those which are rapidly increasing in frequency and severity, also require a visit to the doctor.

What to Expect at the Doctor's Office

The physician will examine the head, eyes, ears, nose, throat, and neck, and also test nerve function. The temperature will be taken. Abnormalities are rarely found. The diagnosis of a headache is usually based on the history given by the patient. If the physician feels that the headache may be "migraine" then an ergot preparation (Cafergot) may be prescribed. Other uncommon types of headaches, such as "cluster headaches, may also be treated with this medicine. However, most headaches are of the tension type, and the basic approach will be that outlined under Home Treatment. Valium is often prescribed for tension headaches because it acts both as a muscle relaxant and as a tranquilizer. Unfortunately, the depression of mental function by this and similar drugs prevents totally successful treatment by tranquilizers.

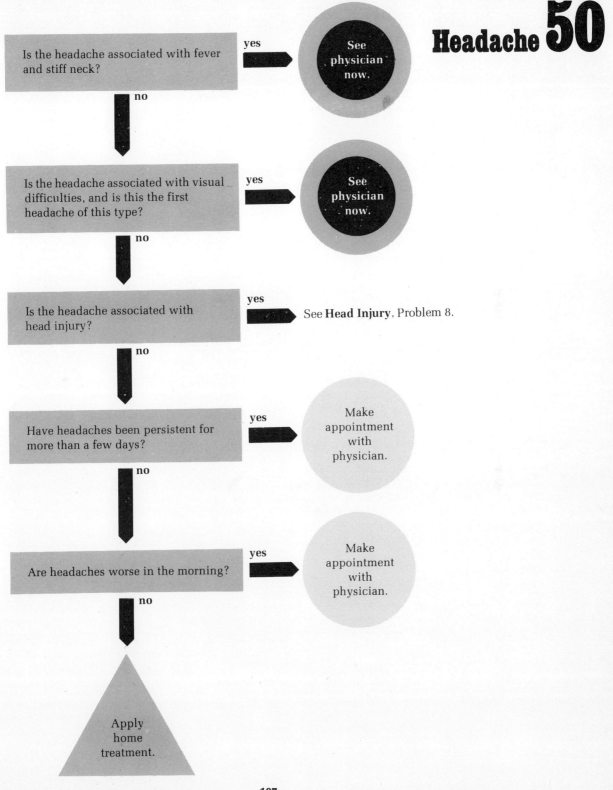

Is the headache associated with fever and stiff neck?

yes → See physician now.

no ↓

Is the headache associated with visual difficulties, and is this the first headache of this type?

yes → See physician now.

no ↓

Is the headache associated with head injury?

yes → See **Head Injury**, Problem 8.

no ↓

Have headaches been persistent for more than a few days?

yes → Make appointment with physician.

no ↓

Are headaches worse in the morning?

yes → Make appointment with physician.

no ↓

Apply home treatment.

J
Chest Pain, Shortness of Breath and Palpitations

51 Chest Pain

Chest pain is a serious symptom meaning "heart attack" to most people. Serious chest discomfort should usually be evaluated by a physician.

However, pain can *also* come from the chest wall (including muscles, ligaments, ribs, and rib cartilage), the lungs, the outside covering of the lungs (pleurisy), the outside covering of the heart (pericarditis), the gullet, the diaphragm, the spine, the skin, and the organs in the upper part of the abdomen. Often it is difficult even for a physician to determine the precise origin of the pain. Therefore, there can be no absolute rules which enable you to determine which pains may be treated at home. The following guidelines usually work and are used by doctors, but there are occasional exceptions.

A shooting pain lasting a few seconds is common in healthy young people, and means nothing. A sensation of a "catch" at the end of a deep breath is also trivial and does not need attention. Heart pain almost never occurs in previously healthy men under 30 years of age or women under 40, and is uncommon for the next 10 years in each sex. Chest-wall pain can be demonstrated by pressing a finger on the chest at the spot of discomfort and reproducing or aggravating the pain. Heart and chest-wall pain are rarely present at the same time. The hyperventilation syndrome (Problem 46) is a frequent cause of chest pain, particularly in young people. If you are dizzy or have tingling in your fingers, suspect this syndrome.

Pleurisy gets worse with a deep breath or cough; heart pain does not. When inflammation of the outside covering of the heart is present, the pain may throb with each heartbeat. Ulcer pain burns with an empty stomach and gets better with food; gallbladder pain often becomes more intense after a meal. Each of these four conditions, when suspected, should be evaluated by a physician.

While heart pain may be mild, it is usually intense. Sometimes a feeling of pressure or squeezing on the chest is more prominent than actual pain. Almost always, the pain or discomfort will be beneath (inside) the breastbone. It may also be felt in the jaw or down the inner part of either arm. There may be nausea, sweating, dizziness, or shortness of breath. When shortness of breath or irregularity of the pulse is present, it is particularly important that a physician be seen immediately. Heart pains may occur with exertion and go away with rest—in this case they are not an actual "heart attack," but are termed "angina pectoris" or "angina."

Home Treatment

You should be able to deal effectively with pain arising from the chest wall. Pain medicines such as aspirin or acetaminophen, topical treatments such as Ben-Gay or Vicks Vaporub, and general measures such as heat and rest should help. If symptoms persist for more than five days, see the physician.

What to Expect at the Doctor's Office

Thorough examination of chest wall, lungs, and heart. Frequently, an electrocardiogram and blood tests. A chest x-ray is usually not helpful and may not be ordered. If the pain remains mysterious, a whole battery of expensive and complex tests may be recommended or required. Pain relief, by injection or by mouth, will sometimes be needed. Hospitalization will be required in instances when the heart is involved or the cause of the pain is not clear.

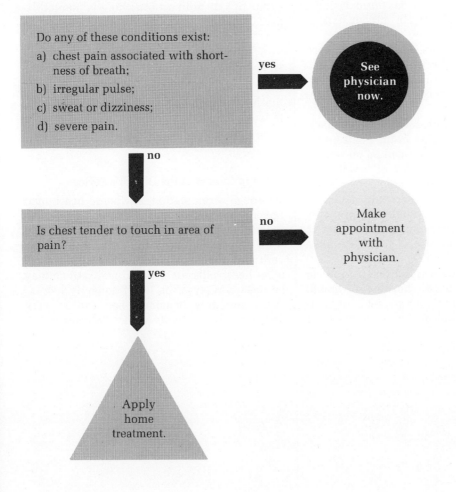

Do any of these conditions exist:

a) chest pain associated with short-ness of breath;

b) irregular pulse;

c) sweat or dizziness;

d) severe pain.

yes → See physician now.

no

Is chest tender to touch in area of pain?

no → Make appointment with physician.

yes

Apply home treatment.

52 Shortness of Breath

When you run hard or climb a hill, you become short of breath. Therefore this symptom is normal under certain circumstances. The medical use of "shortness of breath" does *not* include shortness of breath after heavy exertion, "breathless" with excitement, or having clogged nasal passages. These instances are not cause for alarm.

When you get "winded" after slight exertion or at rest, or wake up in the night out of breath, or have to sleep propped up on several pillows to avoid getting short of breath, you have a serious symptom which should be evaluated promptly by your physician. If wheezing is present, the problem is probably not as serious, but attention is needed just as promptly. In this instance, you may have asthma.

The hyperventilation syndrome (Problem 46) is a common cause of shortness of breath in previously healthy young people and is almost always the problem if the complaint of tingling fingers is present. In this syndrome the patient is actually overbreathing but has the sensation of shortness of breath. A second emotional problem which may present the complaint of difficult breathing is mental depression; deep sighing respirations are a frequent symptom in depressed individuals.

Home Treatment

Rest, relax, use the treatment described for the hyperventilation syndrome (Problem 46), if indicated. If the problem persists, see the physician. There isn't much that you can do for this problem at home.

What to Expect at the Doctor's Office

Thorough examination of lungs, heart, and upper airway passages. Sometimes, electrocardiograms (EKG), chest x-rays, and blood tests. Depending upon the cause and the severity of the problem, hospitalization, fluid pills, heart pills, or asthma medications may be needed. Oxygen is less frequently helpful than commonly imagined, and can be very hazardous for patients with emphysema.

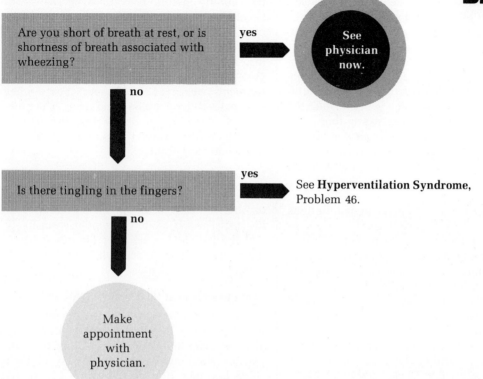

Are you short of breath at rest, or is shortness of breath associated with wheezing?

yes → See physician now.

no ↓

Is there tingling in the fingers?

yes → See **Hyperventilation Syndrome**, Problem 46.

no ↓

Make appointment with physician.

53 Palpita-tions

Everyone gets this one. Pounding of the heart is brought on by strenuous exercise or intense emotion and is seldom associated with serious disease. Most of us have experienced the "bent-bumper syndrome"; after a near collision with another car, the heart seems to almost stop, then pounds with such force that you feel like you're being punched in the chest. Simultaneously, the knees become wobbly and the palms sweaty. These events are due to a large discharge of adrenalin from the adrenal glands. Almost no one is concerned by such pounding of the heart. But if there is no obvious exertion or frightening event, many people become worried.

Most people who complain of palpitations do not have heart disease but are overly concerned about the possibility of such disease and thus overly sensitive to normal heart actions. Often this is because of heart disease in parents, other relatives, or friends.

An irregular or very fast pulse may be more serious. There is a normal variation in the pulse with respiration (faster when breathing in, slower when breathing out). Even though the pulse may speed or slow, the normal pulse has a regular rhythm. Occasional extra heartbeats occur in nearly everyone. Consistently irregular pulses, however, are usually abnormal. The pulse can be felt on the inside of the wrist, in the neck, or over the heart itself. Ask the nurse to check you out on taking pulses on your next visit. Take your own pulse, and those of your family, noting the variation with respiration.

The most common time for palpitations to occur is just before going to sleep. If the pulse rate is under 120, relax.

Hyperventilation may also cause pounding and chest pain, but the heart rate also remains less than 120 beats per minute. Refer to Problem 46.

In adults, a heart rate greater than 120 beats per minute (without exercise) is cause to check with your physician. Young children may have normal heart rates in that range—but they rarely complain of the heart pounding. If one should, check the situation with your physician. Keep in mind that the most frequent causes of rapid heart beat (other than exercise) are anxiety and fever. The presence of shortness of breath (Problem 52) or chest pain (Problem 51) increases the chances of a significant problem.

Home Treatment

If a patient seems stressed or anxious, focus on this rather than upon the possibilities of heart disease. If anxiety does not seem likely and the patient has none of the other symptoms on the chart, discuss it with the physician at your next visit.

What to Expect at the Doctor's Office

Tell the doctor the exact rate of the pulse and whether or not the rhythm was regular. Usually, the symptoms will disappear by the time you see the doctor, so the accuracy of your story becomes crucial. The doctor will examine your heart and lungs. An electrocardiogram (EKG) is unlikely to help if the problem is not present when it's being done. A chest x-ray is seldom needed. Do not expect reassurance from a physician that your heart will be sound for the next month, year, or decade. Your doctor has no crystal ball nor can he or she perform an annual tune-up or oil change. You, not the doctor, are in charge of preventive maintenance of your heart (see Chapters 1 and 2).

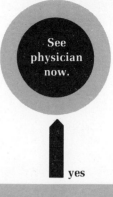

See
physician
now.

Is the pulse consistently irregular, or
is the pulse very rapid (more than 120
beats/minute)?

yes ⟶

Is there shortness of breath, or is there
chest pain?

yes

no

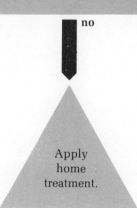

Apply
home
treatment.

no

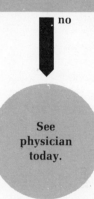

See
physician
today.

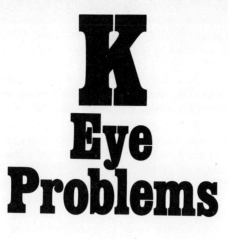

K
Eye Problems

54 Foreign Body in Eye

Eye injuries must be taken seriously. If there is any question, a visit to the physician is indicated. The stakes are too high. A foreign body must be removed, or the threat of infection and loss of sight in that eye is present. Be particularly careful if the foreign body was caused by the striking of metal on metal; this can cause a small metal particle to strike the eye with great force and to penetrate the eyeball.

Under a few circumstances, you may treat at home. If the foreign body was minor, such as sand, and did not strike the eye with great velocity, it may feel like it is still in the eye even when it is not. Small round particles like sand rarely stick behind the upper lid for long.

If it feels like a foreign body is present but it is not, then the cornea has been scraped or cut. A minor corneal injury will usually heal quickly without problems; a major one requires medical attention.

Even if you think the injury to be minor, run through the chart daily. If any symptoms at all are present after 48 hours, and not clearly resolving, see the physician. Minor problems will heal within 48 hours—the eye repairs injury quickly.

Home Treatment

Be gentle. Wash the eye out. Water is good; a weak solution of boric acid is even better if readily available. Inspect the eye yourself and have someone else check it as well. Use a good light and shine it from both the front and the side. Pay particular attention to the cornea—this is a clear membrane which covers the colored portion of the eye. Do not rub the eye—if a foreign body is present you will abrade or scratch the cornea. An eye patch will relieve pain, take it off each day for recheck—usually it is needed for 24 hours or less. Make the patch with several layers of gauze and tape firmly in place—you want some gentle pressure on the eye. Check vision each day—compare the two eyes, one at a time, at reading different sizes of newspaper type from across the room. If you are not sure that all is going well, see the doctor.

What to Expect at the Doctor's Office

Check of vision. Inspection of the eye. Inspection under the upper lid—this is not painful. Usually, a fluorescent stain will be eye-dropped into the eye and the eye will then be examined under ultraviolet light—this is not painful or hazardous. An ophthalmologist (surgeon specializing in diseases of the eye) will examine the eye with a slit lamp. A foreign body, if found, will be removed. In the office, this may be done with a cotton swab, an eyewash solution, or a small needle or "eye spud." If these measures do not suffice, an ophthalmologist may be consulted. An antibiotic ointment is sometimes applied, and an eye patch may be provided. Eye drops which dilate the pupil may be employed. If a foreign body is possibly inside the eye globe, x-rays may be taken.

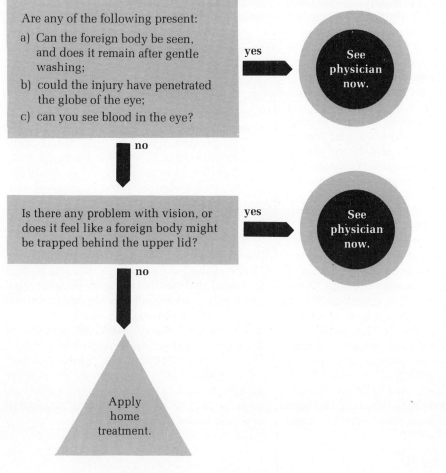

Are any of the following present:

a) Can the foreign body be seen, and does it remain after gentle washing;

b) could the injury have penetrated the globe of the eye;

c) can you see blood in the eye?

yes → See physician now.

no ↓

Is there any problem with vision, or does it feel like a foreign body might be trapped behind the upper lid?

yes → See physician now.

no ↓

Apply home treatment.

55 Eye Pain

Pain in the eye can be an important symptom, and cannot often be safely ignored. Fortunately, it is an unusual complaint. Itching and burning, Problem 57, are more common. Eye pain may be due to injury, to infection, or to an underlying disease. An important disease which can cause eye pain is "glaucoma," which may slowly lead to blindness if not treated. In glaucoma, the fluid inside the eye is under abnormally high pressure, and the globe is tense, causing discomfort. As vision is lost, the first part to go is the lateral vision. Gradually and almost imperceptibly, the field of vision is constricted until the patient has "tunnel vision." In addition, a patient often will see "halos" around lights. Unfortunately, this sequence can occur even when there is no associated pain.

Eye pain is a nonspecific complaint, and questions relating to the pain are often better answered under the more specific headings of Injury (Problem 54), Decreased Vision (Problem 56), or Conjunctivitis (Problem 57). A feeling of tiredness in the eyes, or some discomfort after a long period of fine work (eyestrain) is generally a minor problem and does not really qualify as eye pain. Severe pain behind the eye may result from migraine headaches, and pain either over or below the eye may suggest sinus problems. Pain in both eyes, particularly upon exposure to bright light (photophobia), is common with many viral infections such as flu and will go away as the infection improves. More severe photophobia, particularly when only one eye is involved, may indicate inflammation of the deeper layers of the eye and requires a physician.

Home Treatment

Except for eye pain associated with a viral illness or eyestrain, or minor discomfort which is more tiredness than pain, we do not recommend home treatment. In these instances, resting the eyes, taking a few aspirin, and avoiding bright light may be of help. Follow the chart to the discussion of other problems where appropriate. When symptoms persist, check them out in a routine appointment with your physician.

What to Expect at the Doctor's Office

Check of vision. Check of eye movements. Check of the back of the eye with an ophthalmoscope. An ophthalmologist (surgeon specializing in diseases of the eye) may perform a slit lamp examination. If glaucoma is possible, the doctor may check the pressure of the globe. This is simple, quick, and painless. On occasion, referral to an ophthalmologist. (Many physicians feel uncomfortable with eye symptoms, and referral is common; you may wish to go directly to an ophthalmologist if you have major concern).

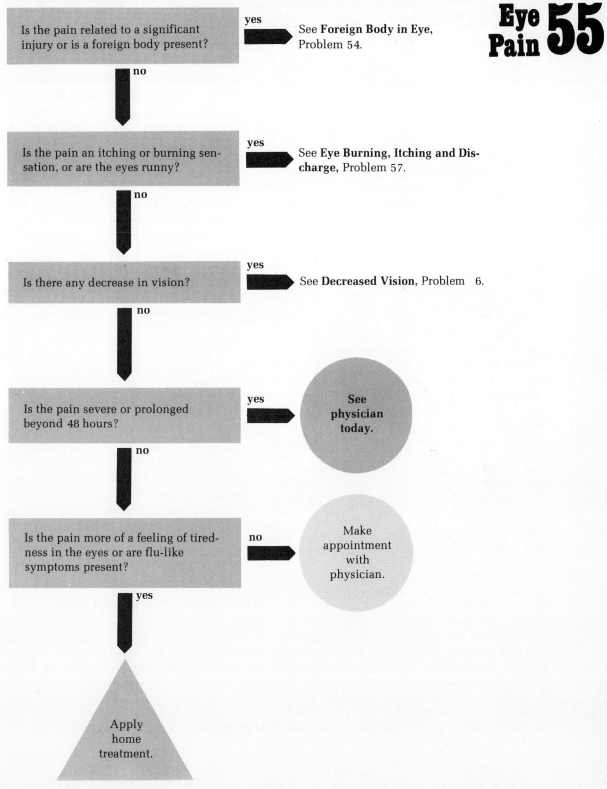

Eye Pain 55

Is the pain related to a significant injury or is a foreign body present?

yes → See **Foreign Body in Eye**, Problem 54.

no

Is the pain an itching or burning sensation, or are the eyes runny?

yes → See **Eye Burning, Itching and Discharge**, Problem 57.

no

Is there any decrease in vision?

yes → See **Decreased Vision**, Problem 6.

no

Is the pain severe or prolonged beyond 48 hours?

yes → **See physician today.**

no

Is the pain more of a feeling of tiredness in the eyes or are flu-like symptoms present?

no → Make appointment with physician.

yes

Apply home treatment.

56 Decreased Vision

Few people need urging to protect their sight. Decrease in vision is a major threat to the quality of life. Usually, professional help is needed. A few syndromes do not require a visit to a health professional. When small, single "floaters" drift across the eye from time to time and do not affect vision, they are not a matter for concern. Slight, reversible blurring of vision may occur after outdoor exposure or with overall fatigue. In young people, sudden blindness in both eyes is commonly a hysterical reaction, and is not a permanent threat to sight; such patients need a doctor but not an eye doctor. After a problem has disappeared it is often impossible to tell what it was; if your problem has reversed itself wait to see if it comes back before seeing the physician.

Usually, the question is not whether to see a health professional, but rather, which one to see. The choice is generally between the ophthalmologist, the optometrist, and the primary-care physician (generalist, internist, or pediatrician). An *optician* does not diagnose eye problems, but dispenses glasses. The *optometrist* is not a physician, but is capable of evaluating the need for glasses, and determining what prescription lens gives the best vision. Conditions well treated by the optometrist are myopia (nearsighted), hyperopia (farsighted), and astigmatism (crooked-sighted). If another disease of the eye is suspected, the optometrist may refer you to an ophthalmologist, who is a highly trained physician and surgeon. The ophthalmologist is the final authority on diseases localized to the eye. Sometimes an eye problem is part of a problem with the general health; in these cases the primary physician is sometimes appropriate.

Try to find the right health professional on the first attempt; this will save you time and money. Eventually, you will be referred to the right person, but it is in your interest to make the process simpler. Following are some examples which usually work, you may have to modify them for your particular situation.

Depending upon the physician manpower in your area the choice will be often different.

- School nurse detects decreased vision in child: ophthalmologist or optometrist—possibly myopia (nearsightedness)

- Sudden blindness in one eye in an elderly person: ophthalmologist or internist—possible stroke or temporal arteritis

- Halos around lights and eye pain: opthalmologist—possibly acute glaucoma (increased pressure in the eye)

- Gradual visual decrease in an adult who wears glasses: ophthalmologist or optometrist—change in refraction of the eye

- Sudden blindness in both eyes in a healthy young person: internist or ophthalmologist—possible hysterical reaction

- Gradual blurring of vision in an older person, not helped by moving closer or farther away: ophthalmologist—possible cataract (scar tissue forming in the lens of the eye)

- Older person who sees far objects best: optometrist or ophthalmologist—presbyopia or farsightedness

- Blurred vision, thirst, large urine output: internist—possible diabetes

- Visual change while taking a medicine: call the prescribing physician—the drug may be responsible

- Decreased vision, one eye, with a "shadow" or "flap" in the visual field: ophthalmologist—possible retinal detachment

What to Expect at the Doctor's Office

Check of vision, eye movements, pupils, back of eye. Eye pressure when indicated, slit lamp examination on occasion. General medical evaluation as required. Refraction to determine a proper corrective lens may be needed; busy ophthalmologists will sometimes refer this procedure to an optometrist. Surgery will be recommended for some conditions.

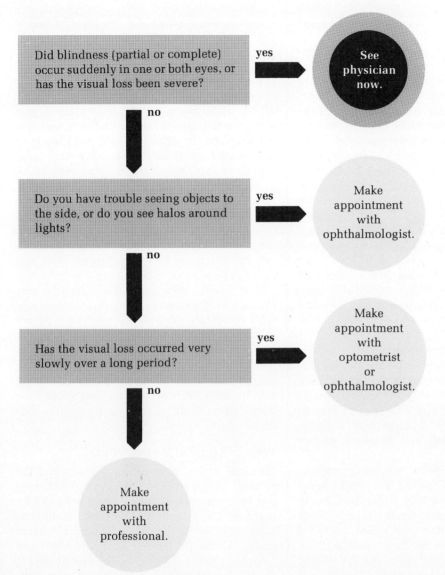

Did blindness (partial or complete) occur suddenly in one or both eyes, or has the visual loss been severe?

yes → See physician now.

no

Do you have trouble seeing objects to the side, or do you see halos around lights?

yes → Make appointment with ophthalmologist.

no

Has the visual loss occurred very slowly over a long period?

yes → Make appointment with optometrist or ophthalmologist.

no

Make appointment with professional.

57 Eye Burning, Itching, & Discharge

These symptoms usually mean "conjunctivitis" or "pink eye," with inflammation of the membrane which lines the eye and the inner surface of the eyelids. The inflammation may be due to an irritant in the air, an allergy to something in the air, a virus infection, or a bacterial infection. The bacterial infections and some of the viral infections (particularly herpes) are potentially serious but are least common.

Many tourists have trouble reading the "Welcome to Los Angeles" sign because of these symptoms. Environmental pollutants in smog can produce burning and itching which sometimes seem as severe as the symptoms experienced in a tear gas attack. These symptoms represent a chemical conjunctivitis, and affect anyone exposed to enough of the chemical. The smoke-filled room, the chlorinated swimming pool, the desert sandstorm, sunglare on a ski slope, or exposure to a welder's arc can give similar physical or chemical irritation.

In contrast, allergic conjunctivitis affects only those certain people who are allergic. Almost always the allergen is in the air, and grass pollens are probably the most frequent offender. Depending upon the season for the offending pollen, this problem may occur in spring, summer, or fall, and usually lasts two to three weeks.

A minor conjunctivitis frequently accompanies a viral cold, giving the well-known symptoms, and lasting only a few days. Some viruses, such as herpes, cause deep ulcers in the cornea and interfere with vision. Bacterial infections cause pus to form, and a thick plentiful discharge runs from the eye. Often the eyelids are crusted over and "glued" shut upon awakening. These infections can cause ulceration of the cornea and are serious.

Some major diseases affect the deeper layers of the eye—those layers that control the operation of the lens and the size of the pupillary opening. This condition is termed "iritis" or "uveitis" and may cause irregularity of the pupil or pain when the pupil reacts to light. Medical attention is required. For true eye pain, see Problem 55. For pain related to injury, see Problem 54.

Home Treatment

If a physical, chemical, or allergic exposure is the cause of the symptoms, there is nothing to do but avoid the exposure. Dark glasses, goggles at work, closed houses and cars with air-conditioning to filter the air, avoidance of chlorinated swimming pools, and other such measures are appropriate. Antihistamines, either over-the-counter or by prescription, may help slightly if the problem is an allergy —but don't expect total relief without a good deal of drowsiness from the medication. Similarly, a viral infection related to a cold or flu will run its course in a few days, and it is best to be patient.

If it doesn't clear up, if the discharge gets thicker, or if you have eye pain or a problem with vision, see your physician. Do not expect a fever with a bacterial infection of the eye; it may be absent. Since the infection is superficial, washing the eye gently will help remove some of the bacteria, but the physician should still be seen. Murine, Visine, and other eyedrops may sooth minor conjunctivitis, but do not cure.

What to Expect at the Doctor's Office

Check of vision, eye motion, eyelids, and the reaction of the pupil to light. An ophthalmologist (surgeon specializing in eye diseases) may perform a slit lamp examination. Antihistamines may be prescribed and general advice given. Antibiotic eyedrops or ointments are frequently given. Cortisone-like eye ointments should be prescribed very infrequently; certain infections (herpes) may get worse with these medicines. If herpes is diagnosed—usually by an ophthalmologist—special eyedrops and other medicines will be needed.

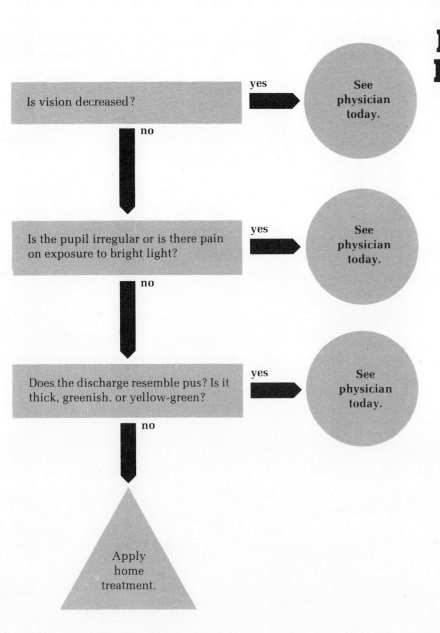

Is vision decreased?

yes → See physician today.

no ↓

Is the pupil irregular or is there pain on exposure to bright light?

yes → See physician today.

no ↓

Does the discharge resemble pus? Is it thick, greenish, or yellow-green?

yes → See physician today.

no ↓

Apply home treatment.

L
The Digestive Tract

58 Nausea, Vomiting, & Diarrhea

Nausea, vomiting, and/ or diarrhea seldom last long. They are common with viral infections (no fever) of the digestive tract. Excess food or alcohol, and/ or minor emotional stresses can also bring them on. As long as they last only for a few days, home treatment is fine; otherwise, see your doctor. An ulcer, gallbladder or intestinal problems, or a serious disease of the digestive tract could be present. Usually not, but it's worth a check.

Even with short-term symptoms, certain additional signs call for a physician, promptly. Suspected bleeding from the digestive tract (other than a little bright blood on the toilet paper—see Problem 62) calls for immediate action. Cramping, intermittent, gas-like pains are usual with diarrhea, but if pain is severe, steady, or prolonged, you may have a more serious problem. If in doubt, call for advice. (See also Abdominal Pain, Problem 60.)

A head injury with repeated nausea and vomiting is potentially serious (Problem 8). In early pregnancy, nausea is common—after the 12th week, it may be cause for concern. In a diabetic, nausea and vomiting may be early signs of a diabetic coma—if the urine tests sugar (and acetone) free, they are *not*. Urinary tract infections which cause these symptoms require medical attention. Many medications cause nausea; some cause diarrhea. If a drug side-effect seems possible, call the prescribing physician.

Dehydration (which is more likely when vomiting and diarrhea are both present) requires a day or so to develop and can usually be avoided. Extreme thirst and dryness of the mouth and tongue suggest dehydration. In infants and children, it can develop more quickly and be more severe. Vomiting all fluids is particularly serious in very small patients since their tolerance is low. As an age guideline: If a child under 2 loses all fluid for as much as 6 hours, between 2 and 6 years old for 8 hours, between 6 and 10 years old for 10 hours, and (anyone) over 10 for 12 hours, call your doctor.

Home Treatment

Avoid solid foods. Don't eat or drink much at one time. Sip clear fluids such as water or ginger ale. Suck on ice chips if nothing else will stay down. Vomiting, diarrhea, and fever increase your need for fluid, so take in as much as comfortable. As the condition improves, add soups, bouillon, jello, and applesauce. Milk products may help, if tolerated, but sometimes aggravate the situation. Work up, slowly, to a normal diet.

Diarrhea responds to these same measures. Applesauce may help slow down the bowel. A tablespoon of Kaopectate after each loose bowel movement will seldom upset the stomach and may help. If Kaopectate is not effective, try Parepectolin or Parelixir.

Recurrent minor bowel problems are common in the United States, possibly due to the lack of fiber in our diets; in countries where high-residue diets are customary, few digestive problems are seen. Your diet should include fresh fruits, vegetables, celery, brans, and whole wheat breads. A tablespoon of Metamucil in water twice daily is a safe, effective (if expensive) way to increase residue.

If symptoms persist beyond 72 hours, contact your physician.

What to Expect at the Doctor's Office

A reasonably complete physical examination, with particular attention to the abdomen; often, blood tests; urinalysis. A plain x-ray of the abdomen is seldom useful but sometimes special x-rays and procedures are needed.

If dehydration is a problem, intravenous fluids and hospitalization may be required for even a self-limited disease. On occasion, surgical treatment is needed.

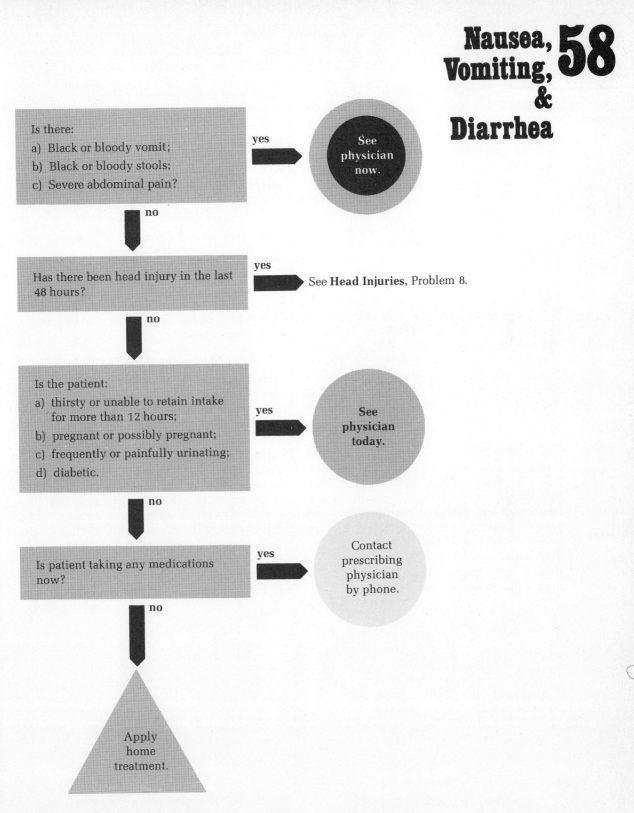

Is there:

a) Black or bloody vomit;

b) Black or bloody stools;

c) Severe abdominal pain?

yes → See physician now.

no

Has there been head injury in the last 48 hours?

yes → See **Head Injuries,** Problem 8.

no

Is the patient:

a) thirsty or unable to retain intake for more than 12 hours;

b) pregnant or possibly pregnant;

c) frequently or painfully urinating;

d) diabetic.

yes → See physician today.

no

Is patient taking any medications now?

yes → Contact prescribing physician by phone.

no

Apply home treatment.

59 Heartburn

Heartburn is irritation of the stomach or of the esophagus, the tube which leads from the mouth to the stomach. The stomach lining is usually protected from the effects of its own acid. But certain factors, such as smoking, caffeine, aspirin, and stress cause this protection to be lost. The esophagus is not protected against acid and a backflow of acid from the stomach into the esophagus causes irritation.

Ulcers of the stomach or the upper bowel may also cause pain. Treatment for ulcers really is the same as for uncomplicated heartburn, provided that pain is not severe and that there is no evidence of bleeding. Vomiting of black, "coffeeground" material or of bright red blood indicates that the time has come to call the doctor. Black stools, rather like tar, have the same significance. (However, iron supplements and bismuth (Pepto-Bismol) will also cause black stools.) Heartburn pain ordinarily does not go through to the back, and such pain may signal involvement of the pancreas or a severe ulcer.

Home Treatment

Avoid substances which aggravate the problem. The most common irritants are coffee, tea, alcohol, and aspirin. The contribution of smoking or stress must be considered in every patient. Relief is often obtained with the frequent (every one to two hours) use of nonabsorbable antacids like Maalox, Mylanta, or Gelusil (see Chapter 7). Antacids should be used with caution by persons with heart disease or high blood pressure because of their high salt content. Sodium bicarbonate or Alka-Seltzer may provide quick relief but are not suitable for repeated use (see Chapter 7). Milk may be substituted for antacid but you usually don't want the calories.

If the pain is worse on lying down, the esophagus is probably the problem. Measures which help prevent the backflow of acid from the stomach into the esophagus should be employed. These are:

- Avoiding reclining after eating.

- Elevation of the head of the bed with four- to six-inch blocks.

- Discontinue the wearing of tight-fitting clothes (girdles, etc.), if applicable.

- Avoid eating or drinking for two hours prior to retiring.

What to Expect at the Doctor's Office

The physician will determine if the problem is due to stomach acid (a peptic acid syndrome). If so, then treatment will be similar to that outlined above. Medications to reduce secretion of acid may be prescribed; none are totally satisfactory. X-rays of the stomach after swallowing barium (upper G.I.) may be done to determine the presence of ulcers and note if backflow of acid from stomach into the esophagus ("hiatal hernia") is present. Since the treatment for any acid syndrome is essentially the same, an x-ray is usually not done on the first visit. Any indication of bleeding will require a more vigorous approach to therapy.

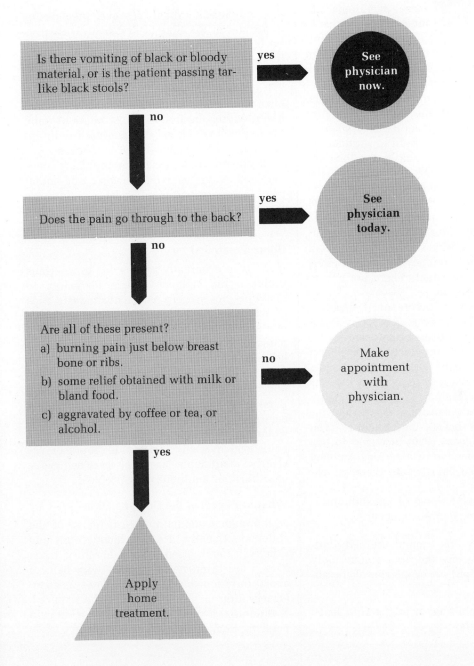

Is there vomiting of black or bloody material, or is the patient passing tar-like black stools?

yes → **See physician now.**

no

Does the pain go through to the back?

yes → **See physician today.**

no

Are all of these present?

a) burning pain just below breast bone or ribs.

b) some relief obtained with milk or bland food.

c) aggravated by coffee or tea, or alcohol.

no → Make appointment with physician.

yes

Apply home treatment.

60 Abdominal Pain

Abdominal pain can be a sign of a serious condition. Fortunately, minor causes for these symptoms are much more frequent.

Although abdominal pain can come from the esophagus, the stomach, the bowel, the female organs, the rectum, the gallbladder, an outpouching of the bowel, or other organs, such pain frequently raises immediate concern about possible appendicitis. Appendix pain usually occurs in the right lower quarter; kidney pain involves the back; the gallbladder—the right upper quarter; the stomach—the upper abdomen; and the bladder or female organs—the lower areas. Exceptions do occur to these rules. Pain from hollow organs (such as the bowel or gallbladder) tends to be intermittent and to resemble gas pains (colic). Pain from solid organs (kidneys, spleen, liver) tends to be more constant. There are exceptions to these rules also.

If the pain is very severe or if bleeding from the bowel is possible, see a physician. Similarly, if there has been a significant recent abdominal injury, see the doctor—a ruptured spleen or other major problem is possible. Pain during pregnancy is potentially serious and must be evaluated; an "ectopic pregnancy" (in the fallopian tube rather than the uterus) can occur before the patient is even aware she is pregnant. Pain localized to one area is more suggestive of a serious problem than is generalized pain (again, there are exceptions).

The most constant signal of appendicitis is the *order* in which symptoms occur:

- Pain—usually first around the belly button or just below the breast bone, only later in the right lower quarter of the abdomen;

- Nausea or vomiting, or at the very least, loss of appetite;

- Local tenderness in the right lower quarter of the abdomen;

- Fever—in the range of 100° to 102°F.

Appendicitis is unlikely if: fever precedes or is present at the time of first pain; if there is *no* fever or a *high* fever (greater than 102°F) in the first 24 hours; if vomiting accompanies or precedes the first bout of pain.

Rupture of the appendix, which is the complication we try to prevent by surgery, is unlikely within the first 18 to 24 hours of pain. Many pains which may be confused with appendicitis will disappear in 6 to 8 hours.

Of course, there are major problems other than appendicitis which cause abdominal pain. Gas pains and minor viral infections are the most common of the various causes. Use the chart to deal with abdominal pain logically.

Home Treatment

If the pain eventually proves due to a serious problem, the stomach should be empty to allow prompt surgery or diagnostic tests. Sips of water or other clear fluids may be taken, but avoid solid foods. A bowel movement, passage of gas through the rectum, or a good belch may give relief—don't hold back. A warm bath helps some patients. The key to home treatment is periodic reevaluation; any persistent pain should be evaluated at the emergency room or the physician's office. Home treatment should be reserved for mild pains which resolve within 24 hours or are clearly identifiable as viral gastroenteritis, heartburn, or another minor problem.

What to Expect at the Doctor's Office

A thorough examination, particularly of the abdomen. Usually, a white blood count and urinalysis, and often other laboratory tests. X-rays are often not important with pain of short duration but are sometimes needed. Observation in the hospital may be required. If the initial evaluation was negative but pain persists, then reevaluation is necessary.

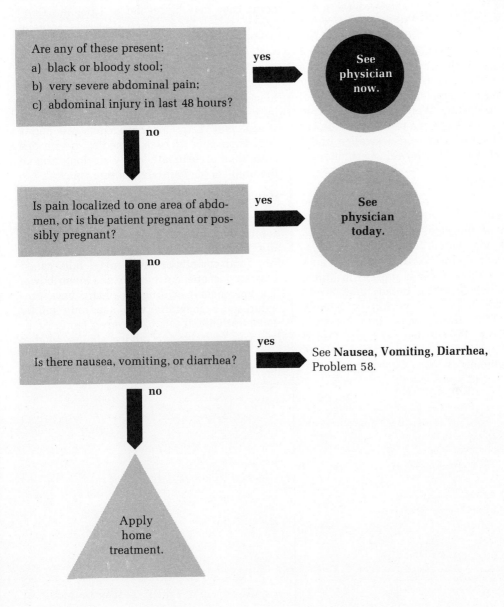

Are any of these present:
a) black or bloody stool;
b) very severe abdominal pain;
c) abdominal injury in last 48 hours?

yes → See physician now.

no

Is pain localized to one area of abdomen, or is the patient pregnant or possibly pregnant?

yes → See physician today.

no

Is there nausea, vomiting, or diarrhea?

yes → See **Nausea, Vomiting, Diarrhea, Problem 58.**

no

Apply home treatment.

61 Constipation

Many patients are preoccupied with constipation. Concern about the shape of the stool, its consistency, its color, and the frequency of bowel movements is often reported to physicians. Such complaints are medically trivial. Only rarely (and then usually in older patients) does a change in bowel habits signal a serious problem. Weight loss and thin pencil-like stools suggest a tumor of the lower bowel. Abdominal pain and a swollen abdomen suggest a possible bowel obstruction.

Home Treatment

We like to encourage a healthy diet for the bowel, followed by a healthy disinterest in the details of the stool elimination process. The diet should contain fresh fruits and vegetables for their natural laxative action and adequate fiber residue. Fiber is present in brans, celery, and whole wheat breads and absent in foods which have been too completely processed. Fiber draws water into the stool and adds bulk, thus it decreases the transit time from mouth to bowel movement and softens the stool.

Bowel movements may occur three times daily or once each three days and still be normal. The stools may change in color, texture, consistency, or bulk without need for concern. They may be regular or irregular. Don't worry about them unless there is a major deviation.

If laxatives are required, we prefer Metamucil, which is a fiber and bulk laxative. Milk of magnesia is satisfactory, but we don't like to see it or stronger traditional laxatives used over a long period. For an acute problem, an enema may help. Fleet's enemas are handy and disposable. If such remedies are needed more than occasionally ask your doctor about the problem on your next routine visit.

What to Expect at the Doctor's Office

If you have had a major change in bowel habits, expect a rectal examination, and usually, inspection of the lower bowel through a long (and sometimes cold) metal tube called a sigmoidoscope. An x-ray of the lower bowel (barium enema) is often needed. These procedures are generally safe and only mildly uncomfortable. If you have only a minor problem you may receive advice similar to that under Home Treatment, without examination or procedures.

Constipation 61

Is constipation associated with:
a) very thin, pencil-like stools,
b) abdominal pain and bloating,
c) weight loss?

yes Make appointment with physician.

no

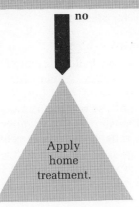

Apply home treatment.

225

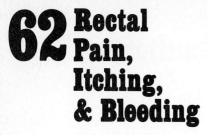

62 Rectal Pain, Itching, & Bleeding

Seldom is a rectal problem major, but the discomfort it can cause may materially interfere with the quality of life, and, unlike most other medical problems, rectal pain does not yield the dividend of a good topic for social conversation.

Hemorrhoids, or "piles," are the most common cause of these symptoms. There is a network of veins around the anus, and they tend to enlarge with age, particularly in individuals who sit a great deal during the day. Straining to have a bowel movement and the passage of hard, compacted stools tends to irritate these veins and they may become inflamed, tender, or clogged. The veins themselves are the "hemorrhoids." They may be external to the anal opening and visible, or they may be inside and invisible. Pain and inflammation usually disappear within a few days or a few weeks, but this interval can be extremely uncomfortable. After healing, a small flap (or "tag") of vein and scar tissue often remains.

Bleeding from the digestive tract is usually serious. We are *not* talking here about the bright red, relatively light bleeding that originates from the hemorrhoids, but blood from higher in the digestive tract which will be burgundy or black. Blood from hemorrhoids may be on the outside of the stool but will not be mixed into the stool substance and frequently will be seen on the toilet paper after wiping. Such bleeding is not medically significant unless it persists for several weeks.

Often a child will suddenly awake screaming in the early evening with rectal pain. This almost always means pinworms. Though these small worms are seldom seen, they are quite common. They live in the rectum, and the female emerges at night and secretes a sticky and irritating substance around the anus into which she lays her eggs. Occasionally, the worms move into the vagina, causing pain and itching in that area. This is not a major problem. It is not well treated in emergency rooms but is a signal to see a physician within a few days. The whole family should be treated to prevent reinfection.

If rectal pain persists more than a week, the physician should be consulted anyway. In such cases, a fissure in the wall of the rectum may have developed, or an infection or other problem may be present.

Home Treatment

Soften the stool, by including more fresh fruits and fiber (bran, celery, whole wheat bread) in the diet, or by use of fiber bulk (Metamucil) or laxatives (milk of magnesia). Keep the area clean. Use the shower as an alternative to rubbing with toilet paper. After gently drying the painful area, apply zinc oxide paste or powder, which will protect against further irritation. The various proprietary hemorrhoid preparations are less satisfactory. We prefer *not* to use compounds with a local anesthetic agent, because these compounds may sensitize and irritate and may prolong healing. Such compounds have a "caine" in the brand name or in the list of ingredients. "Internal" hemorrhoids sometimes may be helped by using a soothing suppository in addition to stool-softening measures. If relief is not complete within a week, see the doctor. Even if the problem resolves quickly, mention it to your doctor on your next visit.

What to Expect at the Doctor's Office

Examination of the anus and rectum. If a clot has formed, the vein may be lanced and the clot removed. Major hemorrhoid surgery is seldom required and should be reserved for the most persistent problems. Usually, advice like that under home treatment will be given.

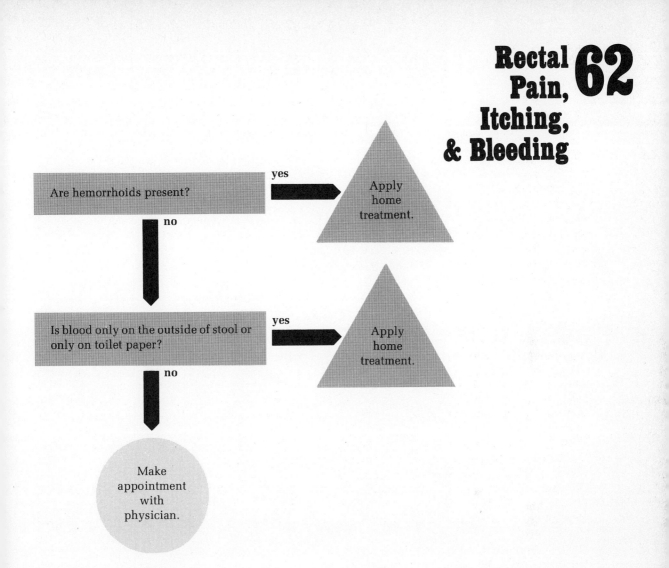

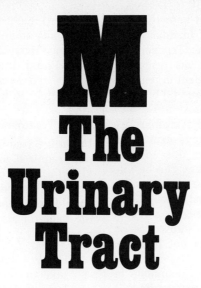

M
The Urinary Tract

63 Painful, Frequent Urination or Blood in Urine (female)

The best-known symptoms of bladder infection are: (1) pain or burning on urination, (2) frequent urgent urination, and (3) blood in the urine.

These symptoms are not always caused by infection due to bacteria. They can be due to a viral infection or to excessive use of caffein-containing beverages (coffee, tea, and cola drinks) or they can have no known cause ("nerves"). When the cause is not bacteria, antibiotics will do no good.

Bladder infection is more common in women than it is in men (most women have it at one time or another) because the female urethra, the tube leading from the bladder to the outside of the body, is only about ½-inch long—a short distance for bacteria to travel to reach the bladder. Sometimes bladder infection is related to sexual activity, hence "honeymoon cystitis" has become a well-known medical syndrome.

Vomiting, back pain, or teeth-chattering, body-shaking chills are not typical of bladder infections and suggest kidney infection. This requires a more vigorous treatment and follow up. A history of kidney disease (infections, inflammations, and kidney stones) also alters the treatment.

Bladder infections are common during pregnancy and may be more difficult to treat. Treatment must, of course, take the pregnancy into account.

Some physicians have developed procedures by which a patient with these symptoms may obtain a urinalysis without first seeing the physician. If the urinalysis indicates a possible bacterial infection, the patient is seen and appropriate therapy begun. If this is not the case, then the patient is directed to use home treatment for 24 hours. If there is no relief during that time, the patient is then seen.

It is quite possible that many bacterial bladder infections will respond to home treatment alone. Still it makes good sense to use antibiotics when appropriate and this has become standard medical practice. Antibiotics may be especially important in recurrent bladder infections. Even if you are inclined towards doing without drugs, you should see the doctor unless the symptoms respond quickly and completely to home treatment.

Home Treatment

Definitive treatment of a urinary tract infection requires an antibiotic (which may not alter the symptoms for 24 hours). Quicker relief is afforded by home treatment which should be started immediately (although all of the bacteria may not be eliminated by these measures).

- Drink a lot of fluids: Increase fluid intake to the maximum (up to several gallons of fluid in the first 24 hours). Bacteria are literally washed from the body during the resulting copious urination.

- Drink fruit juices: Putting more acid into the urine, while less important than the quantity of fluids, may help bring relief. Cranberry juice is the most effective, as it contains a natural antibiotic.

Begin home treatment as soon as symptoms are noted. For women with recurrent problems, an important preventive measure is to wipe the toilet tissue from front to back (*not* back to front) following urination. Most bacteria which cause bladder infections come from the rectum.

What to Expect at the Doctor's Office

A urinalysis and culture should be performed. The back and abdomen are usually examined. In women with a discharge, an examination of both the vagina and the discharge is often necessary. With preexisting kidney disease or symptoms of kidney infection, a more detailed history and physical are needed and extra laboratory studies may be necessary.

If urinary tract infection is proved, an antibiotic should be prescribed. Gantrisin or Ampicillin are the most commonly used unless there is an allergy. Tetracycline is also used frequently, but should not be given to pregnant women or young children.

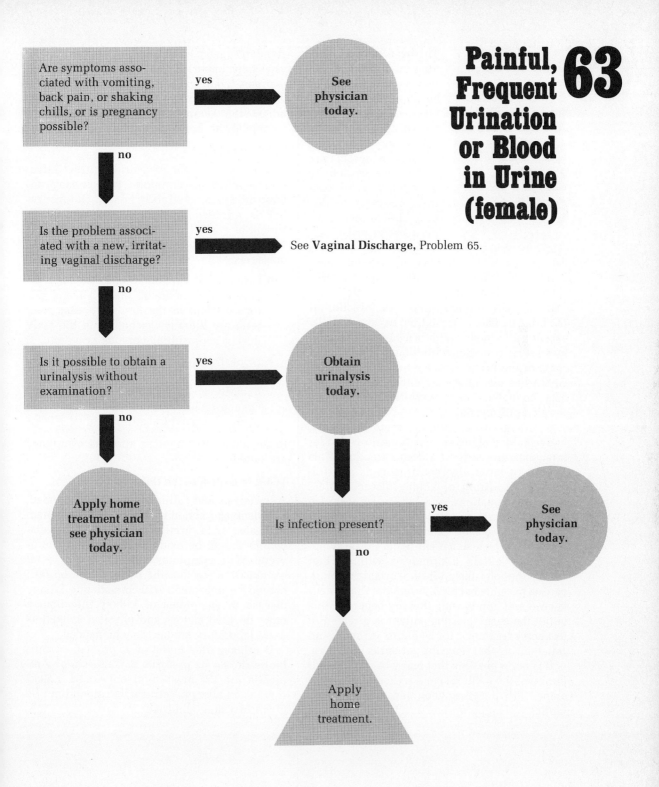

Are symptoms asso-
ciated with vomiting,
back pain, or shaking
chills, or is pregnancy
possible?

yes → See physician today.

no

Is the problem associ-
ated with a new, irritat-
ing vaginal discharge?

yes → See **Vaginal Discharge,** Problem 65.

no

Is it possible to obtain a
urinalysis without
examination?

yes → Obtain urinalysis today.

no

Apply home treatment and see physician today.

Is infection present?

yes → See physician today.

no

Apply home treatment.

Painful, 63 Frequent Urination or Blood in Urine (female)

63 Painful, Frequent Urination or Blood in Urine (male)

The best-known symptoms of bladder infection are: (1) pain or burning on urination, (2) frequent urgent urination, and (3) blood in the urine.

These symptoms are not always caused by infection due to bacteria. They can be due to a viral infection or to excessive use of caffein-containing beverages (coffee, tea, and cola drinks), or they can have no known cause ("nerves"). When the cause is not bacteria, then antibiotics will do no good.

In males with these symptoms, infection of the prostate gland (prostatitis) or venereal disease is quite likely. With prostatitis, difficulty in starting urination, dribbling, or decreased force of the urinary stream are often present. Gonorrhea discharges are milky and thick but may be noted only intermittently (refer to Problems 62 and 66).

Vomiting, back pain, or teeth-chattering, body-shaking chills are not typical of bladder infections and suggest kidney infection. This requires a more vigorous treatment and follow up. A history of kidney disease (infections, inflammations, and kidney stones) also alters the treatment.

Some physicians have developed procedures by which a patient with these symptoms may obtain a urinalysis without first seeing the physician. If the urinalysis indicates a possible bacterial infection, the patient is seen and appropriate therapy begun. If this is not the case, then the patient is directed to use home treatment for 24 hours. If there is no relief during that time, the patient is then seen.

It is quite possible that many bacterial bladder infections will respond to home treatment alone. Still it makes good sense to use antibiotics when appropriate and this has become standard medical practice. Antibiotics may be especially important in recurrent bladder infections. Even if you are inclined towards doing without drugs, you should see the doctor unless the symptoms respond quickly and completely to home treatment.

Home Treatment

Definitive treatment of a urinary tract infection requires an antibiotic (which may not alter the symptoms for 24 hours). Quicker relief is afforded by home treatment which should be started immediately (although all of the bacteria may not be eliminated by these measures).

- Drink a lot of fluids: Increase fluid intake to the maximum (up to several gallons of fluid in the first 24 hours). Bacteria are literally washed from the body during the resulting copious urination.

- Drink fruit juices: Putting more acid into the urine, while less important than the quantity of fluids, may help bring relief. Cranberry juice is the most effective, as it contains a natural antibiotic.

Begin home treatment as soon as symptoms are noted.

What to Expect at the Doctor's Office

A urinalysis and culture should be performed. The back and abdomen are usually examined. In males with urethral discharge, the discharge should be examined under the microscope. With symptoms of prostatitis, a rectal examination (so that the prostate can be felt) should be expected. With preexisting kidney disease or symptoms of kidney infection, a more detailed history and physical as well as extra laboratory studies may be needed.

If urinary tract infection is proved, an antibiotic should be prescribed. Gantrisin or Ampicillin are the most commonly used, unless there is an allergy. Tetracycline should not be given to young children.

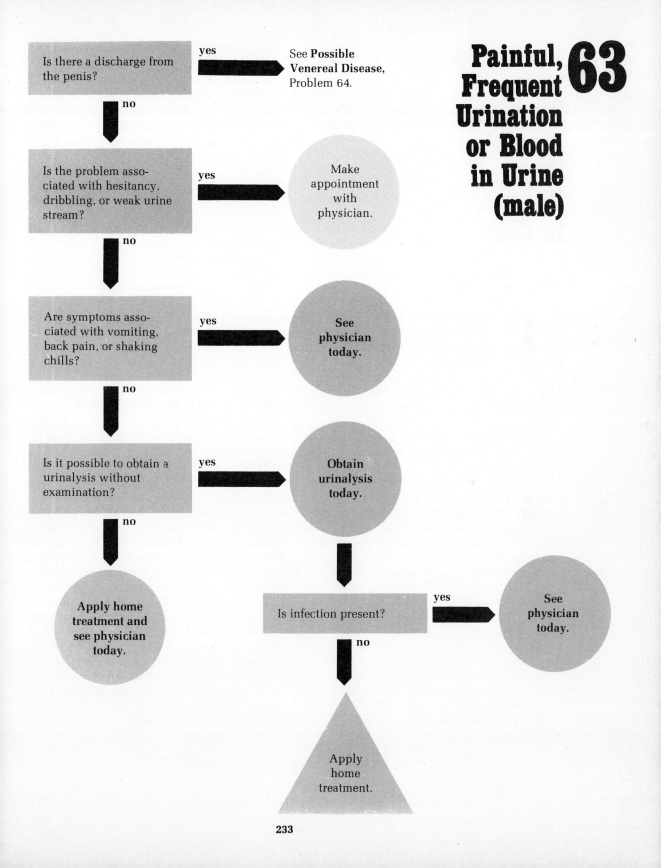

Is there a discharge from the penis?

yes → See **Possible Venereal Disease**, Problem 64.

no ↓

Is the problem associated with hesitancy, dribbling, or weak urine stream?

yes → Make appointment with physician.

no ↓

Are symptoms associated with vomiting, back pain, or shaking chills?

yes → **See physician today.**

no ↓

Is it possible to obtain a urinalysis without examination?

yes → **Obtain urinalysis today.**

no ↓

Apply home treatment and see physician today.

Is infection present?

yes → **See physician today.**

no ↓

Apply home treatment.

Painful, Frequent Urination or Blood in Urine (male)

63

64 Discharge from Penis or Possible Venereal Disease in Men

A venereal disease is any disease which is transmitted by sexual contact but the term "VD" usually refers to gonorrhea or syphilis. Seldom are these diseases spread by means other than sexual contact, since the organisms do not survive for long outside the body.

Gonorrhea (the clap, the strain) causes a discharge from the penis. Primary symptoms, burning and pain on urination and a thick, mucous discharge, start within 2 to 14 days of exposure. If not treated, the patient may note difficulty in urinating, fever, and pain, tenderness, and swelling of the testicles. Repeated infections may result in sterility or in a scarred urethra which requires surgical dilatation, a most unpleasant procedure. Following possible exposure, symptoms such as discharge, sore throat, rash or a hot, swollen joint require medical consultation.

Syphilis has three distinct phases. *Primary syphilis* may result in a small, painless ulcer (chancre) on the genitalia (occasionally on the mouth or hands) which appears ten to ninety days after sexual contact with an infected person. If untreated, the chancre will heal in approximately four to six weeks. The patient is highly infectious during the primary stage. In about 30 percent of all male cases, there is no chancre and thus no sign of this phase. *Secondary syphilis* occurs shortly after the first stage (although it occasionally occurs simultaneously with the chancre). This stage is a rash which may have small bumps, flat red lesions, or may, in fact, take almost any form except blisters. It is especially likely to involve the soles, palms, and face. The *tertiary* stage occurs years later. This is the bad stage in which people die or go insane. Tertiary syphilis may affect virtually any part of the body, but death usually comes from involvement of the heart or nervous system.

Persons who have had sexual contact with individuals infected with syphilis or gonorrhea must be contacted so that adequate therapy may be given. Public health departments often provide free care. Unnecessary consequences can be avoided.

Home Treatment

Don't treat at home with left-over or borrowed medicines. You won't do it right. If you've got it, think you might have it, or have been exposed to it, see the doctor.

The use of condoms does offer some but not total protection from venereal disease. Urination immediately following intercourse appears effective in reducing the probability of gonorrhea, the problem of having intercourse when your bladder is full notwithstanding. The usefulness of antibiotics given prior to exposure (as in the military) is questionable.

What to Expect at the Doctor's Office

A diagnosis of gonorrhea is confirmed by testing a culture from the discharge (or from the infected throat or joints) for gonococcus bacteria. The gonococcus is seldom cultured from the genital tract if there is no discharge. Examination of the discharge under the microscope tentatively differentiates between gonorrhea and so-called "nonspecific urethritis," which, though it is probably a venereal disease, has no known serious long-term effects. Gonorrhea is usually treated with penicillin injections; nonspecific urethritis is often treated by giving tetracycline by mouth.

In all cases of suspected venereal disease, a blood test for syphilis should be obtained. (In many states this is required to obtain a marriage license. However, since the test does not become positive for from three weeks to three months after exposure, any negative test during that period must be repeated when the three months has elapsed.

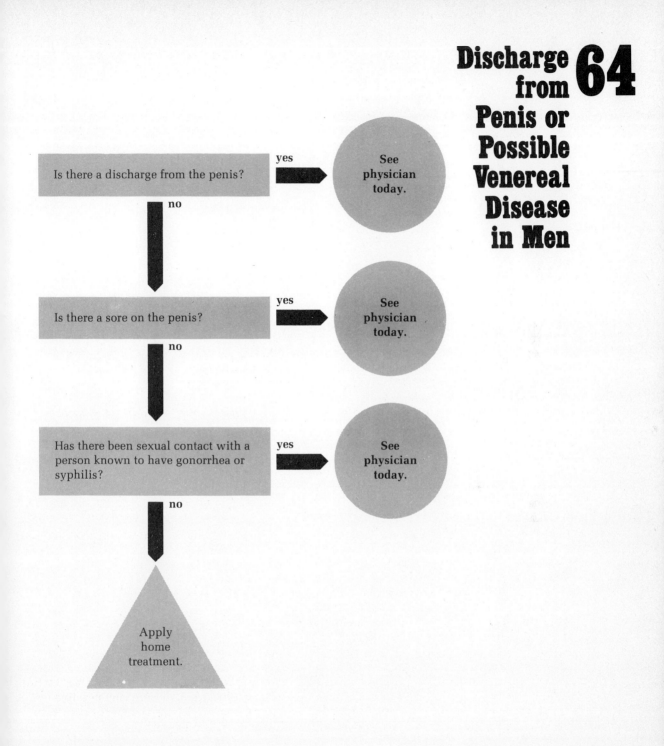

Is there a discharge from the penis? — yes → See physician today.

no

Is there a sore on the penis? — yes → See physician today.

no

Has there been sexual contact with a person known to have gonorrhea or syphilis? — yes → See physician today.

no

Apply home treatment.

Discharge from Penis or Possible Venereal Disease in Men 64

N
For
Women Only

HOW TO DO A BREAST SELF-EXAMINATION

Most lumps in the breast are not cancer. Most women will have a lump in a breast at some time during their life. Many women's breasts are naturally lumpy (so-called "benign fibrocystic disease"). Obviously every lump or possible lump cannot and should not be subjected to surgery.

Cancer of the breast does occur, however, and is best treated early than later. Regular self-examination of your breasts gives you the best chance of avoiding serious consequences. Self-examination should be monthly, just after the menstrual period.

The technique is as follows:

- First, examine your breasts in the mirror, first with your arms at your side and then with both arms over your head. The breasts should look the same. Watch for any change in shape or size, or for dimpling of the skin. Occasionally a lump which is difficult to feel will be quite obvious just by looking.

- Next, while lying flat, examine the left breast using the inner finger tips of the right hand and pressing the breast tissue against the chest wall. Do not "pinch" the tissue between the fingers; all breast tissue feels a bit lumpy when you do this. The left hand should be behind your head while you examine the inner half of the left breast and down at your side when you examine the outer half. Do not neglect the part of the breast underneath the nipples or that which extends outward from the breast toward the underarm. A small pillow under the left shoulder may help.

- Repeat this process on the opposite side.

Any lump detected should be brought to the attention of your physician. Regular self-examination will tell you how long it has been present and whether it has changed in size. This information is very helpful in deciding what to do about the lump; even the doctor often has difficulty with this decision. Self-examination is an absolute necessity for a woman with naturally lumpy breasts; she is the only one who can really know whether a lump is new, old, or has changed size. For all women, regular self-examination offers the best hope that surgery will be performed when, and only when, it is necessary.

THE GYNECOLOGICAL EXAMINATION

Examination of the female reproduction organs, usually called a "pelvic" examination, may be expected for complaints related to these organs and in conjunction with the annual "Pap" smear. This examination yields a great deal of information and often is absolutely essential for diagnosis. By understanding the phases of the examination and your role in them, you can make it possible for an adequate examination to be done quickly and with a minimum of discomfort.

Positioning: Lying on your back, put your heels in the stirrups (the nurse will often assist in this step). Move down to the very end of the examination table, with knees bent. Get as close to the edge as you can. Now let your knees fall out to the sides as far as they will go. Do not try to hold the knees close with the inner muscles of the thigh. This will tire you and make the examination more difficult.

The key word during the examination is "relax"; you may hear it several times. The vagina is a muscular organ and if the muscles are tense, a difficult and uncomfortable examination is inevitable. You may be asked to take several deep breaths in an effort to obtain relaxation. We hope that understanding what is happening will also help you relax.

External examination: Inspection of the labia, the clitoris and vaginal opening is the first step in the examination. The most common findings are cysts in the labia, rashes, and so-called "venereal warts." These problems have effective treatments or may need no treatment at all.

Speculum examination: The speculum is the "duck-billed" instrument used to spread the walls of the vagina, so that the inside may be seen. It is *not* a clamp. It may be constructed of metal or plastic. The plastic ones will "click" open and closed, don't be alarmed. Contrary to popular opinion, the speculum is not stored in the refrigerator. Usually they are warmed before use.

If a Pap smear or other test is to be made, the speculum examination usually will come before the finger (manual) examination and the speculum will be lubricated with water only. A lubricant or a manual examination may spoil the test. If these tests are not needed, then the manual examination may come first. The speculum also opens the vagina so that insertion of an intrauterine device (IUD) or other procedures can be done.

Manual examination: By inserting two lubricated, gloved fingers into the vagina and pressing on the lower abdomen with the other hand, the physician can feel the shape of the ovaries and uterus as well as any lumps in the area. The accuracy of this examination depends on the degree of relaxation of the patient and the skill of the physician. Fat women cannot be examined as well; this is another good reason not to be overweight. Usually, the best pelvic examinations are done by those who do them most often. You need not require a gynecologist, but be sure that your internist or family practitioner does "pelvics" on a regular basis before you request a yearly gynecology exam. The nurse practitioner who does pelvic examinations regularly is usually expert also. The Pap smear alone does *not* require a great deal of experience and is the single most important part of the examination.

Many physicians will also perform a rectal or rectovaginal (one finger in rectum and one in vagina) examination. These examinations can provide additional information.

If you are nervous about the pelvic examination, ask the physician to explain what is going on during the examination. Usually there is a drape over your knees and the physician sits on a stool out of your line of sight. You can cooperate better if you understand the procedures, and you will feel less awkward during this examination if you and the physician are communicating effectively.

The "Pap" Smear

Since the Pap test is of unique importance to women, you should be familiar with the basics of this procedure. As explained above, a scraping of the cervix and a sample of the vaginal secretions is obtained with the aid of a speculum. This provides cells for study under the microscope. A trained technician (a cytologist) can then classify the cells according to their microscopic characteristics. There are five classes: Class I and II are negative for tumor cells; Class III and IV are suspicious but not definite for tumors; Class V is definite for tumors. If your smear is Class III or IV, your physician will ask you to return for another pap test or a biopsy of the cervix. This does not mean that cancer is definite. If your smear is Class V, your physician will explain the approach to confirming the diagnosis and starting treatment.

The Pap smear is our most effective tumor-finding test for two reasons. First, a single test detects approximately 90 percent of the most common cancers of the womb and 70 to 80 percent of the second most common. Second, both these common types of cancer grow slowly; current evidence indicates that it may take 10 years or more for a single focus of cancer of the cervix to spread. Thus there is an excellent chance that regular Pap smears will detect the cancer before it spreads. Although Pap smears are usually done annually, this is not magical, and an argument can be made for longer intervals. Cancer of the cervix is rare under the age of 25. Pap smears are usually begun at that age. However, cancer of the cervix is more frequent with moderate-to-heavy sexual activity, especially if there are multiple partners, and probably regular Pap testing should begin when regular sexual activity begins. There is almost no evidence that the use of birth control pills requires more frequent Pap smears.

65 Vaginal Discharge

Discharge from the vagina is common. Most of the many possible causes require the physician. If the discharge is slight, doesn't hurt or itch, and is not cheesy, smelly, or bloody, and if there is no possibility of a venereal disease and the patient is past puberty, the problem may be observed at home—for a time.

Abdominal pain suggests the possibility of serious disease, ranging from gonorrhea to an ectopic pregnancy in the fallopian tube. Bloody discharge between periods, if recurrent or significant in amount, suggests much the same. Discharge in a girl before puberty is rare and should be evaluated.

If sexual contact in the past few weeks might possibly have resulted in a venereal disease, the physician *must* be seen. Do not be afraid to take this problem to the doctor, and be frank in naming your sexual contacts, for their own benefit. Information will be kept confidential and you will not be embarrassed by the physician, who will have confronted this situation many times.

Monilia is a fungus which may infect the walls of the vagina and cause a white, cheesy discharge. Trichomonas is a common microorganism which can cause a white frothy discharge and intense itch. A mixture of bacteria may be responsible for a discharge, so-called non-specific vaginitis. These infections are not serious and do not spread to the rest of the body, but are bothersome. They will sometimes but not always go away by themselves. If discharge persists beyond a few weeks, make an appointment with the physician.

In older women, lack of hormones can cause "atrophic" vaginitis. Prescription creams are sometimes needed if symptoms are bothersome. Foreign bodies, particularly a forgotten tampon, are a surprisingly frequent cause of vaginitis and discharge.

Home Treatment

Hygiene and patience are the home remedies. If you have a discharge, douche daily (and following intercourse) with a Betadine solution (2 tablespoons to a quart of water) or baking soda (one teaspoon to a quart). If you are taking an antibiotic such as tetracycline for some other condition; call your physician for advice on changing medication. If the discharge persists despite treatment for more than two weeks, or becomes worse, see the physician. Do not douche for 24 hours prior to seeing the physician. Some physicians will prescribe over the phone for a vaginitis. Multipurpose medications (AVC, Sultrin Creams) or those active against yeast (Mycostatin, Vanobid, Candeptin) are useful in this situation.

What to Expect at the Doctor's Office

Pelvic examination. If a venereal disease is suspected, culture of the mouth of the womb (cervix) is mandatory. If not, examination of the discharge under the microscope or culture of the discharge is sometimes but not always needed. Suppositories or creams are the usual treatment. If venereal disease is at all likely, antibiotics (usually penicillin) will be prescribed. Oral medication for fungus or trichomonas may be used in severe cases. The sexual partner(s) may require treatment as well.

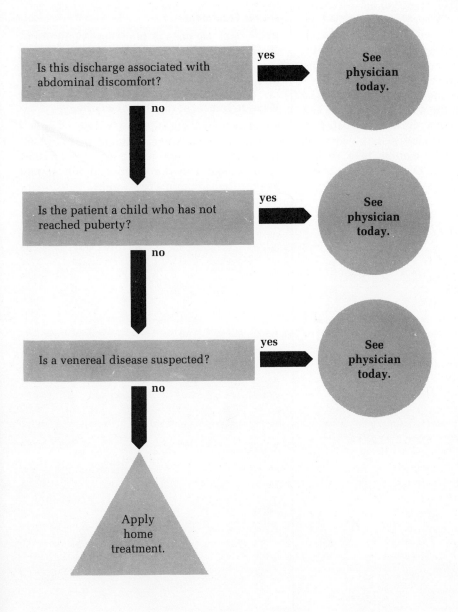

Is this discharge associated with abdominal discomfort?

yes → See physician today.

no

Is the patient a child who has not reached puberty?

yes → See physician today.

no

Is a venereal disease suspected?

yes → See physician today.

no

Apply home treatment.

66 Bleeding between Periods

Most often, the interval between two menstrual periods is free of bleeding or spotting. Many women experience such bleeding, however, even though no serious condition is present. Women with an intrauterine birth control device (IUD) are particularly likely to have occasional spotting. If bleeding is slight and occasional, it may be ignored. Serious conditions such as cancer and abnormal pregnancy may be first suggested by bleeding between periods. So if bleeding is severe or occurs three months in a row, a physician must be seen. Often a serious problem can be detected best when the bleeding is not active. The gynecologist or the family physician is a better resource than the emergency room. Any bleeding after the menopause should be evaluated by a physician.

Home Treatment

Relax, and use pads or tampons. Avoid use of aspirin if possible; in theory, it may prolong the bleeding. If in doubt about the effect of other medicines, call your doctor.

What to Expect at the Doctor's Office

Some personal questions, a pelvic examination, and a "pap" smear should be expected. If bleeding is active, pelvic examination and "pap" smear may be postponed but should be performed within a few weeks.

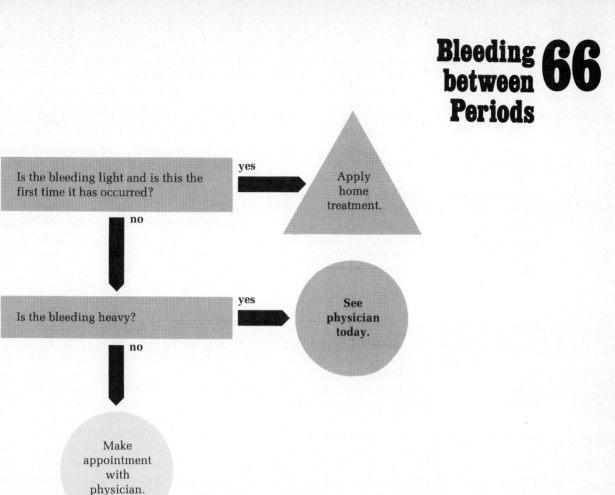

Is the bleeding light and is this the first time it has occurred?

yes → Apply home treatment.

no

Is the bleeding heavy?

yes → See physician today.

no

Make appointment with physician.

67 Difficult Periods

Adverse mood changes and fluid retention are very common in the several days prior to the menstrual period. Such problems are vexing and can be difficult to treat, but are a result of normal hormonal variations during the menstrual cycle.

The menstrual cycle is different for different women. Periods may be regular, irregular, light, heavy, painful, painfree, long, or short, and still be normal. Variation in the menstrual cycle is medically less significant than bleeding, pain, or discharge between periods. Only when problems are extremely severe or recur for several months is medical attention required. Emergency treatment is seldom needed.

Home Treatment

We do not believe that diuretics (fluid pills) or hormones are frequently indicated. Perhaps this is callous. Still, as we have said in other sections of this book, we prefer the simple and natural to the complex and artificial. Following hormone treatment, all too frequently we have seen mood changes which are worse than the premenstrual tension, as well as potassium loss, gouty arthritis, and psychological drug dependency from diuretics.

Salt tends to hold fluid in the tissues and to cause edema. The most natural diuretic is to cut down on salt intake. In the United States the typical diet has ten times the required amount of salt; many authorities feel that this is one cause of high blood pressure and arteriosclerosis. No matter how hard you try to eliminate salt from your diet, you will still have more than enough. If you can eliminate some salt, you may have less edema and fluid retention. If food tastes flat without salt, try using lemon juice as a substitute. The commercial salt substitutes are also satisfactory. Products with the word "sodium" or the symbol "Na" anywhere in the list of ingredients contain salt.

For menstrual cramps, aspirin. Products claimed to be designed for menstrual cramps (e.g., Midol) have aspirin as the main ingredient. Many patients swear by such compounds, and they are fine if you want to pay the premium. But we don't understand, on a scientific basis, why they should be any better than plain aspirin.

What to Expect at the Doctor's Office

Advice. Frequently, diuretics or hormones by prescription. Pelvic examination is often unrewarding and sometimes may not be performed. In cases of heavy bleeding, a "D and C" may be required. Hysterectomy should not be performed for this complaint alone. If a tumor is found, surgery will sometimes be needed, but the common "fibroid" tumor will often stop growing by itself and surgery may not be needed. Such tumors often grow slowly and stop growth at the menopause, so that by waiting, an operation can be avoided. If the "Pap smear" is positive, however, surgery is often indicated.

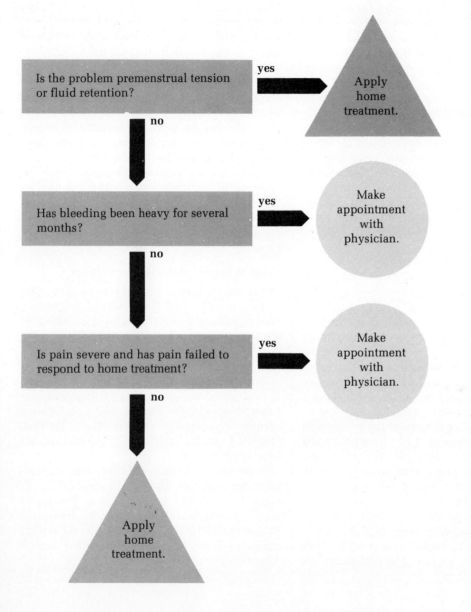

68 Possible Venereal Disease in Women

VD. Clap. Gonorrhea. GC. Whites. Strain. PID. Syphilis. Lues. Chancre. Sores. These are terms for venereal disease. VD is not for home treatment, and, if VD is suspected, you must contact a physician. These conditions require antibiotic treatment after accurate diagnosis, and sexual contacts must be treated to prevent spreading.

Do *not* attempt to use antibiotics that you have at home or can buy in the street for these serious infections. You do not know the potency, the dose, or the duration of treatment required, and we are not going to tell you. Tragedies from inadequate home treatment include sterility, heart infection, death from ectopic pregnancy, and needless infection of others.

There are two main venereal diseases, gonorrhea and syphilis, and of the two, gonorrhea is considerably more common than syphilis. In women, infection with either disease is often hard to determine, since it is "inside" rather than "outside." A vaginal discharge may be dismissed for several months until gonorrhea infection has moved to the fallopian tubes, the joints, or into the bloodstream. Gonorrhea is painful as well as dangerous. The male partner with gonorrhea may report "clap," "whites," or "strain"; all common names for gonorrhea or "GC". In syphilis, the male may report a "sore" on the penis (see Problem 62). The sore on the woman is often not noticed. An unexplained skin rash (on the body and including the palms and soles) occurs several weeks after the infection and indicates the secondary stage of the disease.

"Crabs," "lice," "trich," and several other conditions may be spread by sexual exposure, but are more often transmitted by nonvenereal routes. Don't force any unreasonable accusations on your partner when one of these are found. Only syphilis and gonorrhea are invariably transmitted by sexual contact. When recent experience includes oral or anal sex, either syphilis or gonorrhea may be found infecting the mouth or the rectum.

Home Treatment

Hygiene after sexual contact is of potential benefit. Douche thoroughly after the encounter if suspicious or worried. Inspection of the penis during foreplay for sores or white thick discharge is useful for the uncertain situation. In the world's "oldest profession," such inspection is routinely practiced. A condom or "rubber" is a reasonably effective barrier to disease transmission. Thus home treatment consists of *prevention*. After infection, or after possible infection, you need a doctor.

What to Expect at the Doctor's Office

Pelvic examination and treatment. For gonorrhea, a culture of the mouth of the womb. For syphilis a blood test and a scraping of the sore. Venereal disease (VD) clinics are available in most large cities and provide high-quality service at little or no cost.

Your sexual contacts *must* be treated, even if they have no symptoms, for they can continue to spread the disease and can develop serious complications themselves. Do not withhold names. Treatment of contacts is discreetly performed.

Treatment is with antibiotics, usually penicillin by injection. Be sure to mention an allergy to penicillin to the doctor. Treatment with the program recommended by the United States Public Health Service is almost always curative—but you can catch another dose a few days later. Be prepared.

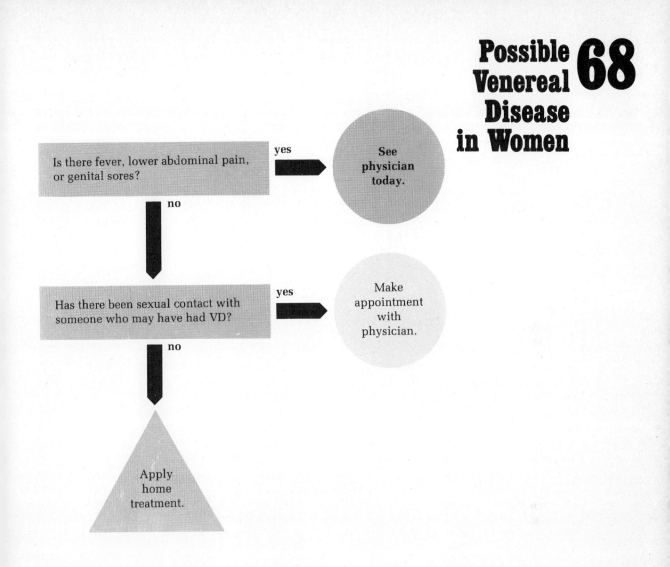

Is there fever, lower abdominal pain, or genital sores?

yes → See physician today.

no ↓

Has there been sexual contact with someone who may have had VD?

yes → Make appointment with physician.

no ↓

Apply home treatment.

O
Sexual Problems

Sex is an area in which we all experience some insecurity. Every individual has anxieties and fears; everyone thinks that friends and colleagues are free from such problems. There are no personal experts in sex. No personal experience can constitute both a broad sampling of individual differences and probe the depths of a long-standing, profoundly intimate relationship. Since everyone knows his or her own activities, and for the most part imagines what others are doing, myths abound.

Each generation and most individuals discover anew the exhilaration of a good sexual experience. In a perverse game played between the generations, a variety of contradictory rules for the conduct of sexual relationships are dogmatically advocated. Accusations are formulated, anxieties created, and health disturbed.

Good feelings are what sex is all about. But the good feelings go beyond the pleasurable physical sensations of sexual arousal. Feeling good about yourself, about your partner, about intimacy—these are the good feelings you need for sex to be its most satisfying and pleasurable. A number of factors may prevent these good feelings; only a minority of these are related to sexual function itself. Anxiety or depression from any cause may result in problems with sex. Attitudes toward sex do create problems, usually unnecessarily. We are particularly concerned with an emerging view of the sexual partner as an orgasm machine, with a preoccupation with technique rather than feeling, and with the resulting depersonalization of the sexual relationship.

Anxiety about sex, especially in the learning stage, must be counted as normal simply because it is a universal phenomenon. This anxiety has been compounded by both of the two dominant contemporary approaches toward sex. The first approach considers sex as an unspeakable subject. Moralistic

251

and Victorian, it wages a whispering war against sexual feelings and seeks to cover the notion of intimate pleasure with a blanket of guilt. It seeks to enforce a code of behavior through fear. This attitude is hardly conducive to resolution of anxiety or to the dissolution of ungrounded sexual fears.

Secondly, since the Kinsey Report there has been an increasing trend toward the regarding of sex as a competitive sport, with score kept according to the number of partners, number of orgasms achieved, and number of positions used. Popular writers who tell when, where, and how to do it, have placed emphasis upon performance and technique. Portions of the women's movement and of the youth movement have been exploited. Technique is only a part of sexual satisfaction. Fear of failure to perform is no less damaging than fear of unwanted pregnancy, fear of not getting married, or fear of venereal disease. Fear of impotence is the chief cause of impotence. Fears of inadequate arousal are not conducive to maximal pleasure.

The new anxieties about sex, voiced to us with increasing frequency in the past several years, can be traced to this conflict. Sex is commercially promoted, in caricature, as a game played with tape measure and stop watch. Standards are established which are at the same time fictitious and undesirable, and the new anxieties result from failure to achieve the "standards."

We have no secret solutions to sexual problems. As in other portions of this book, we are attempting to restate some common sense concepts known to most readers but commonly neglected in considering health. Together with a few medical facts, we hope this will enable you to deal more effectively and realistically with your problems. In the following paragraphs we briefly consider the sexual issues of masturbation, sexual fantasies, virility, premature ejaculation, impotence, turn-ons, orgasm, and sexual variety. Many other sources provide more detailed treatment of these complicated subjects.

Masturbation is a common practice in both men and women. It is an outlet for tensions when there is no opportunity for other sexual practices. Self-stimulation is not a disease, and causes no physical harm to the body. It does not cause warts, pimples, sterility, or feeblemindedness. We often encounter patients deeply disturbed about this practice and whose guilt concerning it pervades other portions of their lives. The only frequent problem with masturbation is guilt over the practice.

There are no human beings past puberty who do not have *sexual fantasies*. The content of such fantasies is widely variable. Seduction, exploitation, and sadomasochism are common elements, as well as softer and more romantic themes. Individuals frequently have a favorite and recurring sexual fantasy. Sexual surrogates are common fantasies; they may be Robert Redford or Raquel Welch, or they may be persons who are a part of the individual's everyday life. If the fantasy contains unacceptable elements such as violence or sexual relations with a sibling or parent, then there is often some distress concerning the meaning of the fantasy. Sexual fantasies, like masturbation, are a form of release of sexual tensions. They are almost never complicated by subsequent illegal or perverse activity. Imagination is a gift. With all of the thinking of matters sexual, it is natural that fantasies develop. A feature of the human mind is that fantasies cannot be suppressed by thinking about them. If you avoid guilt about your fantasies, you promote your sexual health.

Virility is another major myth. We frequently encounter patients with fears that their sexual activity is too frequent or too infrequent. Part of this problem stems from publication of average figures from large-scale sex surveys. People who find their practices distant from the averages often are concerned. Relax. It may be eight times a day or eight times a year. The only rule worth remembering is that in a stable relationship, the frequency of sexual activity should be a workable compromise between the desires of the partners.

Another area of anxiety concerns the *sexual equipment.* Men worry about the size of their penis. Women worry that their breasts are too big or too small, their legs too fat or too thin. Men worry about a pigeon-chest, no hair on their chest, or too much hair on their chest. Women are concerned that their hair does not properly frame their face, that they have hairs around the nipples, or that their total image is too dowdy or too awkward or too cheap. There is little that is worthwhile in such concerns.

Some individuals are more attractive than others. In the dimension of sensuality, some are more sensual than others. However, the breadth of taste runs from Rubens to Twiggy. Somebody likes you the way you are. Men may like large women or slender women who wear clothes well. Women may be excited by broad shoulders or by a thoughtful gesture. Whether this whole business is due to cultural indoctrination or to innate differences between the sexes, the point is the same. Usually, the sexual equipment is the least important part of the problem! If you fear that you were not created the most attractive of creatures to the opposite sex, you will find that this difficulty can be reduced by warmth, affection, and humanity. In sex, how you feel *about* each other is more important than how you feel *to* each other.

The man frequently worries unnecessarily about penis size. In point of fact, there is little difference in size of the erect penis between different men, although there are significant differences in the resting state. Moreover, the vaginal canal, which accommodates birth, is potentially much larger than the thickest of penises. The size and rigidity of the penis will vary for the same man at different times. Some factors affecting erect penile size are physical, such as the length of time since previous intercourse; and some are psychological. Impotence is seldom due to disease of genitalia, nerves, or blood vessels. No male is equally potent at all times, and all males are, on some occasions, impotent. Chronic impotence implies chronic anxiety, at least partially compounded by worry over the impotence.

Premature ejaculation, while physically the opposite of impotence, has the same cause. Again, relaxation is usually a solution. There are some other potential aids. A firm pinch on the tip of the penis will delay ejaculation. A condom (rubber) usually will decrease sensation for the male so that ejaculation is delayed. Seldom are such measures necessary for more than a few occasions.

Female orgasm is the most written-about sexual phenomenon of recent years. This subject has been linked inseparably to aspects of the women's movement. It has been pointed out that some women are multi-orgasmic, and may climax several times during a single coupling. It has been held that equality of orgasm is a principal requirement for sexual equality. On the other hand, it has been observed that a large number of women, probably a majority, do not have orgasms with regularity. The emerging sexual myth is that these women, although a majority, are in some way abnormal. In point of fact, many women relating a deep and satisfactory sexual experience over many years do not report frequent orgasms during that experience. If you let others tell you what you should be doing, and then allow guilt to develop when you don't meet false "norms," you are promoting these myths. Of all human activities, the sexual should be directed by the individual, at his or her own pace and style.

A variety of sexual practices have been recently reemphasized. These include "swinging," group sex, sex with the aid of various appliances, and sex in a virtual infinity of positions. Such practices are recorded in all eras of human literature, but advocates of sexual variety were discouraged by legal and ethical barriers until recently. Medically, there is no reason either to encourage or discourage sexual variety and experimentation. The problems presently seen are a reaction to earlier attitudes. People now feel guilty that their sex life has insufficient variety. For example, the majority of heterosexual activity takes place in the "male-superior" position. This position is often the most satisfactory for both partners, since it allows the deepest penetration and the sensitivity value of being face to face. Recent derogation of this technique as the "missionary position" illustrates ignorance of history and anatomy; the accusatory tone of the phrase suggests an attempt to arouse guilt and anxiety about a normal practice.

Other individuals, for equally good reasons, prefer many different positions, or find their greatest satisfactions with a particular alternative technique. There is no right way and no standard pattern for sexual expression. Averages are meaningless in a personal relationship between two individuals. Such relationships may be physically expressed in a wide variety of ways, none of which have any superiority to the others. You have personal freedom to be either ordinary or exotic—with pleasure, and without guilt.

Sex is not a competitive sport. Sexual health, for the great majority of individuals, reduces to common sense. If it feels good to both partners, do it. If it doesn't feel good, don't do it. Don't allow the fear of being "hung-up" to become the major hang-up. Individuals should not allow other individuals, equally nonexpert, to define their satisfaction for them; there remain "different strokes for different folks."

Section III

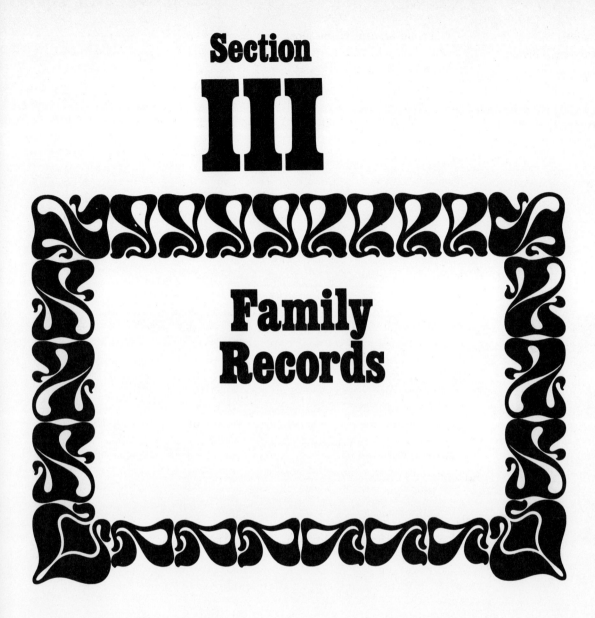

Family Records

Immunizations

DPT = Diphtheria, Pertussis (Whooping Cough), and Tetanus (Lockjaw)

DT = Diphtheria and Tetanus (Lockjaw)

Polio = Oral Polio

Measles = Measles Vaccine

Mumps = Mumps

Rubella = German Measles (Three Day Measles

Name: _____ _____ _____ _____ _____ _____

Recommended Age:	Date	Date	Date	Date	Date	Date
2 months						
DPT #1						
Polio #1						
4 months						
DPT #2						
Polio #2						
6 months						
DPT #3						
Polio #3						
12 months						
Measles						
Mumps						
Rubella						
18 months						
Polio Booster						
DPT Booster						
5 Years						
Polio Booster						
DPT Booster						

Others

_____ _____ _____ _____ _____ _____

_____ _____ _____ _____ _____ _____

_____ _____ _____ _____ _____ _____

_____ _____ _____ _____ _____ _____

Note: Diphtheria and Tetanus is recommended every 10 years for life, with an additional tetanus booster for contaminated wounds more than 5 years after the last booster.

Childhood Diseases

Whooping Cough

Name	Date	Place	Remarks

Chicken Pox

Name	Date	Place	Remarks

Measles

Name	Date	Place	Remarks

Mumps

Name	Date	Place	Remarks

German Measles (Rubella)

Name	Date	Place	Remarks

Other Diseases:

_____

_____ _____ _____ _____
_____ _____ _____ _____
_____ _____ _____ _____
_____ _____ _____ _____
_____ _____ _____ _____

_____

_____ _____ _____ _____
_____ _____ _____ _____
_____ _____ _____ _____
_____ _____ _____ _____
_____ _____ _____ _____

_____

_____ _____ _____ _____
_____ _____ _____ _____
_____ _____ _____ _____
_____ _____ _____ _____

_____

_____ _____ _____ _____
_____ _____ _____ _____
_____ _____ _____ _____
_____ _____ _____ _____
_____ _____ _____ _____

Family Medical Information

Name	Blood type	RH Factor	Allergies (including drug allergies)
_____	_____	_____	_____
_____	_____	_____	_____
_____	_____	_____	_____
_____	_____	_____	_____
_____	_____	_____	_____
_____	_____	_____	_____
_____	_____	_____	_____

Hospitalizations

Name   Date   Hospital
_____   _____   _____

Address   Reason
_____   _____

Name   Date   Hospital
_____   _____   _____

Address   Reason
_____   _____

Name   Date   Hospital
_____   _____   _____

Address   Reason
_____   _____

Name   Date   Hospital

_____   _____   _____

Address   Reason

_____   _____   _____

Name   Date   Hospital

_____   _____   _____

Address   Reason

_____   _____   _____

Name   Date   Hospital

_____   _____   _____

Address   Reason

_____   _____   _____

Name   Date   Hospital

_____   _____   _____

Address   Reason

_____   _____   _____

Name   Date   Hospital

_____   _____   _____

Address   Reason

_____   _____   _____

Name   Date   Hospital

_____   _____   _____

Address   Reason

_____   _____   _____

Name   Date   Hospital

_____   _____   _____

Address   Reason

_____   _____

Name   Date   Hospital

_____   _____   _____

Address   Reason

_____   _____

Name   Date   Hospital

_____   _____   _____

Address   Reason

_____   _____

Name   Date   Hospital

_____   _____   _____

Address   Reason

_____   _____

Name   Date   Hospital

_____   _____   _____

Address   Reason

_____   _____

Name   Date   Hospital

_____   _____   _____

Address   Reason

_____   _____

Index

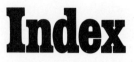

Where multiple page references are listed, the most detailed discussion is indicated by boldface numbers, where applicable.